DATE DUE

9/16/85		APR 24 1989
MAY 25 1987		
APR 10 1988		
11/1/88 York Hosp.		
Due 7.5.92		

OXFORD MEDICAL PUBLICATIONS

Mental illness in pregnancy and the puerperium

Mental illness in pregnancy and the puerperium

EDITED BY

MERTON SANDLER

Professor of Chemical Pathology,
Institute of Obstetrics and Gynaecology
(University of London)

Oxford
OXFORD UNIVERSITY PRESS
New York Toronto
1978

Oxford University Press, Walton Street, Oxford OX2 6DP

OXFORD LONDON GLASGOW NEW YORK
TORONTO MELBOURNE WELLINGTON CAPE TOWN
IBADAN NAIROBI DAR ES SALAAM LUSAKA ADDIS ABABA
KUALA LUMPUR SINGAPORE JAKARTA HONG KONG TOKYO
DELHI BOMBAY CALCUTTA MADRAS KARACHI

© Oxford University Press 1978

ISBN 0 19 261150 X

British Library Cataloguing in Publication Data

Mental illness in pregnancy and the puerperium. —
    (Oxford medical publications).
    1. Pregnancy — Psychological aspects — Congresses
    2. Puerperium — Psychological aspects — Congresses
    I. Sandler, Merton   II. Series
    618.3   RG588   78-40805

ISBN 0-19-261150-X

Typeset by Hope Services, Wantage
Printed in Great Britain
by Billings & Sons Ltd., Guildford and Worcester

Foreword

PROFESSOR SIR JOHN DEWHURST

The disorders of mind during pregnancy have received far less attention than the disorders of the body. In the past this was of course appropriate since the physical risks the mother and child ran were very great. With the increasing safety of childbearing, it might have been thought that much more attention would have been focused on the mental disorders of the pregnant state. This has not happened, however, although there has been much greater interest shown in the emotional aspects of pregnancy in general.

Perhaps the relative neglect of mental illness related to childbearing can be explained by the need for co-operation between two groups of specialized doctors with—outwardly at least—little in common. It would not be exaggerating to say that neither understands the other's problems to any great extent. In each field, moreover, there have been of late scientific, as distinct from purely clinical, advances which have made interdisciplinary co-operation even more difficult.

The symposium on mental illness in pregnancy, labour, and the puerperium on which this book is based was therefore an unusually important one in that it represented one of the relatively few recent attempts to assemble experts from each field to tackle some of the problems and to do so in depth. The symposium was a highly successful one and it is hoped that it will lead not only to immediate benefits but also to more co-operative studies in this area and further scientific discoveries in the future.

Contents

Contents

List of contributors

C. BREWER
Department of Psychiatry, University of Birmingham, and British Pregnancy Advisory Service, Austy Manor, Wootton Wawen, Solihull, West Midlands B95 6DA.

I. F. BROCKINGTON
Department of Psychiatry, The University Hospital of South Manchester, West Didsbury, Manchester M20 8LR.

A. COPPEN
Medical Research Council Neuropsychiatry Laboratory, West Park Hospital, Epsom, Surrey KT19 8PB.

J. L. COX
University Department of Psychiatry (Royal Edinburgh Hospital), Morningside Park, Edinburgh EH10 5HF.

SIR JOHN DEWHURST
Institute of Obstetrics and Gynaecology, Queen Charlotte's Hospital, Goldhawk Road, London W6 0XG.

P. DONNELLY
Department of Psychiatry, The University Hospital of South Manchester, West Didsbury, Manchester M20 8LR.

M. GELDER
University Department of Psychiatry, The Warneford Hospital, Oxford OX3 7JX.

D. HARVEY
Institute of Obstetrics and Gynaecology, Queen Charlotte's Hospital, Goldhawk Road, London W6 0XG.

C. HYDE
Lecturer in Psychiatry, University of Manchester

R. E. KENDELL
University Department of Psychiatry (Royal Edinburgh Hospital, Morningside Park, Edinburgh EH10 5HF.

R. KUMAR
Institute of Psychiatry, Department of Psychiatry, De Crespigny Park, Denmark Hill, London SE5 8AF.

List of contributors

P. J. LEWIS
Institute of Obstetrics and Gynaecology, Queen Charlotte's Hospital, Goldhawk Road, London W6 0XG.

C. H. NAYLOR
Central Middlesex Hospital, Acton Lane, London NW10 7NS.

BRICE PITT
Psychogeriatric Unit, The London Hospital, 2a Bow Road, London E3 4LL.

R. PRIEST
Department of Psychiatry, St. Mary's Hospital, Harrow Road, London W9 3RL.

KAY ROBSON
Institute of Psychiatry, Department of Psychiatry, De Crespigny Park, Denmark Hill, London SE5 8AF.

M. SANDLER (editor)
Bernhard Baron Memorial Research Laboratories, Department of Chemical Pathology, Queen Charlotte's Maternity Hospital, Goldhawk Road, London W6 0XG.

E. M. SCHOFIELD
Department of Psychiatry, University of Manchester, West Didsbury, Manchester M20 8LR.

G. STEIN
Maudsley Hospital, Denmark Hill, London SE5 8AZ.

K. WOOD
Medical Research Council Neuropsychiatry Laboratory, West Park Hospital, Epsom, Surrey KT19 8PB.

Introduction

B. PITT

Our current interest in mental illness in pregnancy and the puerperium is nothing new, but follows a long tradition wherein psychiatrists have been intrigued by women who break down at the time of childbearing. Hamilton wrote an excellent monograph entitled *Post-partum psychiatric problems* which was published in St. Louis in 1962. His survey of the nineteenth-century literature on puerperal and 'lactational' psychoses, listing 300 references, is unrivalled, and his tribute to the remarkable treatise by Marcé, published in Paris in 1858 entitled *Traité de la folie des femmes enceintes, des nouvelles accouchés et des nourrices* is especially gracious and well merited. When Marcé wrote, it was believed that these puerperal and lactational psychoses were specific entities, unlike other mental illnesses and occurring only at these times, but early in the twentieth century, Bleuler (1911) stated that schizophrenia presenting post-partum had no special features and Kraepelin (1913) stated that puerperal mania was only provoked by childbirth when already latent. Then in 1926 Strecker and Ebaugh, after studying a series of 50 cases of mental illness in the puerperium, concluded that as all could be classified as manic depressive psychosis, toxic-exhaustive psychosis, or schizophrenia, there was no such entity as 'post-partum psychosis'. Pugh, Jerath, Schmidt, and Reed (1963) demonstrated that women are actually more liable to be admitted to psychiatric wards, especially for affective illness, in the first three months post-partum. Several controlled studies (e.g. Seager 1960) have shown the importance of constitutional factors in such serious psychiatric breakdown. In their heredity, previous psychiatric history, and premorbid personalities post-partum psychotics are far more like other psychotic women than like puerperal women free from psychosis.

Thomas and Gordon (1959) advanced three hypotheses about the part childbirth plays in causing psychosis:

1

Introduction

(1) Childbirth is a source of significant stress originating in physical factors such as hormonal disturbance or haemorrhage, or in psychological factors which can cause external stress, such as that produced by an unwanted pregnancy, or internal stress, such as that produced by difficulty in adjusting to the maternal role.

(2) Childbirth is just one of any number of possible precipitants against a background of a constitution, inherited or acquired, which predisposes to psychosis indistinguishable from that unrelated to childbirth.

(3) There is a personality or physical defect in these patients, relating specifically to sexual and reproductive life (i.e. an 'Achilles' heel hypothesis).

Evidence exists to support all three hypotheses. The fact of the increased admission rate after childbirth bears out the 'significant event' theory, though as the importance of obvious physical factors and external psychological stress seems small, the mother's internal conflicts may be more critical. However Gordon and Gordon (1960) and Brown, Bhrolcháin, and Harris (1975) have suggested that social factors, such as poor housing and 'having so many children one doesn't know what to do', may be important. The similarity of post-partum psychotics to other psychotic women supports the second hypothesis. The 'Achilles' heel' is almost an extension in my view of the importance of psychological conflict in the first. The anecdotal but plausible studies from the Cassell Psychiatric Hospital (Hayman 1962; Lomas 1959, 1960; Daniels and Lessow 1964) and the Tavistock Clinic (Douglas 1963), suggest the relevance of an obsessional, compliant, conformist, sensitive, controlled *personality*, whose defences against primitive feelings are threatened by closeness to that very primitive creature, a baby, and *marriage* to a passive dominant husband, and intense mutual dependency of husband and wife. Taking a more organic view, Dalton (1977) has claimed that women who get depressed post-partum are sensitive to progesterone deficiency and exhibit euphoria towards the end of pregnancy but a subsequent tendency to the premenstrual syndrome.

2

Introduction

There have been remarkably few prospective or community studies in the literature; the vast bulk of papers concerned women admitted to psychiatric hospital in the throes of psychosis. Two general practitioner surveys, however, by Ryle (1964) and Tod (1964) showed an incidence of postpartum depression of 3 per cent, far in excess of the 0·1–0·2 per cent generally agreed for admissions with post-partum psychosis. Such depression was evidently less severe than psychosis though much more of a problem than the trifling, transitory, and usual 'third day blues' (Pitt 1973). Since then several studies in this country (Pitt 1968; Dalton 1971; Rees and Lutkins 1971) and in Scandinavia (Nilsson, Kaij, and Jacobson 1967) have shown that moderate states of depression, which the mother finds unusual and troublesome, develop after as many as 10 per cent of deliveries and may last for months or even for more than a year. Other such studies are now in progress, notably by Kumar and Robson (Chapter 4).

Pregnancy is rightly being given more attention. It is as interesting to speculate on the dearth of psychiatric admissions at this time as on the excess in the puerperium. This deficit hardly seems matched by a lack of the milder manifestations of emotional disturbance in pregnancy. A generally raised level of anxiety, specific fears of foetal abnormality and of the impending delivery, mood swings lasting from minutes to weeks, and cravings and aversions (Trethowan and Dickens 1972) have all been reported (Pitt 1965; Rees 1971), to say nothing of the psychogenic factor in some cases of hyperemesis. The major hormonal changes of pregnancy are perhaps as relevant to these disturbances as the obvious psychological and social implications. The tendency for these symptoms to subside very quickly after delivery could be related in part to the sudden fall in hormone concentrations to pre-pregnancy levels, though relief at being safely delivered seems a more obvious factor. It is an intriguing paradox that although the majority of mothers are so relieved, a substantial minority feel no better or decidedly worse and that psychiatric morbidity therefore actually increases in the puerperium.

3

Introduction

Is it the hormones or the baby, now out of the womb and demanding attention, or is it both? The almost universal 'third day blues' could represent a brief spell of hormonal imbalance as levels of oestrogen and progesterone subside, but is easily comprehensible as an anti-climax; after the joy and satisfaction of having pushed the baby out into the world comes the realization that he has to be fed and changed and comforted. Breast feeding difficulties are especially prominent in the early days.

Does the setting of the delivery make much difference? There are those who claim that the 'medicalization of motherhood' in hospital creates emotional problems, and that 'third day blues' are unknown after confinements at home. It was said that my own finding that almost 11 per cent of women who had their babies at the London Hospital were depressed at the time of the post-natal examination six weeks later (Pitt 1968) could be explained by my dealing with a teaching hospital clientele, though in fact none of the factors associated with delivery in a teaching hospital—primiparity, previous complications, or being a doctor, a doctor's wife, or a nurse—was significantly associated with puerperal depression. How important is bonding, or the lack of bonding, between mother and baby, in determining maternal emotions? Klaus, Jerauld, Kreger, McAlpine, Steffa, and Kennel (1972) have shown the effects of close contact between mother and baby on subsequent maternal behaviour; is this support for the Leboyer (1975) technique of delivery, which sets aside some time for the mother to stroke her newly met infant and for recognition and reunion outside the womb? What about fathers? Does their greater involvement in the delivery alter their attitude to mother and baby? It seems likely. The phenomenon of 'engrossment' by fond fathers after active involvement in their baby's birth has been described by Greenberg and Morris (1974). Is this of any relevance to maternal mental illness?

Finally, there is the important topic of the treatment of established mental illness and of the effects of drugs given during pregnancy on the foetus. It is reassuring to have learnt (Savage 1978) that psychotropic drugs given to the lactating mother appear only in very small quantities in her breast milk. Their effects on the foetus in pregnancy are discussed in Chapter 10.

References

Bleuler, E. (1911). *Dementia praecox or the group of schizophrenias* (trans. J. Zinkin, 1950). International Universities Press, New York.

Brown, G. W., Bhrolcháin, M. N., and Harris, T. (1975). *Sociology* 9, 225.

Dalton, K. (1971). *Br. J. Psychiat.* 118, 689.

—— —— (1977). *The premenstrual syndrome and progesterone therapy.* Heinemann, London.

Daniels, R. S. and Lessow, H. (1964). *Psychosomatics* 5, 21.

Douglas, G. (1963). *Br. J. med. Psychol.* 36, 271.

Gordon, R. E. and Gordon, K. K. (1960). *Obstet. Gynaec.* 15, 433.

Greenberg, M. and Morris, N. (1974). *Am. J. Orthopsychiat.* 44, 520.

Hayman, A. (1962). *Br. J. med. Psychol.* 35, 135.

Hamilton, J. A. (1962). *Post-partum psychiatric problems.* C. V. Mosby, St. Louis.

Klaus, M. H., Jerauld, R., Kreger, N., McAlpine, W., Steffa, M., and Kennel, J. H. (1972). *New Engl. J. Med.* 280, 460.

Kraepelin, I. (1913). *Lectures on clinical psychiatry* (3rd English edn.). Bailliere, Tindall, and Cassel, London.

Leboyer, F. (1974). *Birth without violence.* Wildwood, London.

Lomas, P. (1959). *Br. J. med. Psychol.* 32, 117.

—— (1960). *Br. J. med. Psychol.* 33, 61; 105.

Marcé, L. V. (1858). *Traité de la folie des femmes enceintes des nouvelles accouchés et des nourrices.* Bailliere, Paris.

Nilsson, A., Kaij, L., and Jacobson, L. (1967), *J. psychosom. Res.* 11, 327; 341.

Pitt, B. (1966). *A study of emotional disturbance associated with childbearing with particular reference to depression arising in the puerperium.* MD Thesis, University of London.

—— (1968). *Br. J. Psychiat.* 114, 1325.

—— (1973). *Br. J. Psychiat.* 122, 431.

Pugh, R., Jerath, B. K., Schmidt, W. M., and Reed, R. B. (1963). *New Engl. J. Med.* 268, 1224.

Rees, W. D. and Lutkins, S. G. (1971). *J. Roy. Coll. gen. Practit.* 21, 26.

Ryle, A. (1964). *J. ment. Sci.* 107, 279.

Seager, C. P. (1960). *J. ment. Sci.* 106, 214.

Savage, A. L. (1978). *Br. J. Psychiat.* 132, 200.

Strecker, E. A. and Ebaugh, F. G. (1926). *Arch. Neurol.* 15, 239

Thomas, C. L. and Gordon, J. E. (1959). *Am. J. ment. Sci.* 238, 363.

Trethowan, W. J. and Dickens, G. (1972). In *Modern perspectives in*

Introduction

psycho-obstetrics ed. J. G. Howells, pp. 251–68. Oliver and Boyd, Edinburgh.

Tod, E. D. M. (1964). *Lancet* ii, 1264.

Introduction

R. G. PRIEST

It is commonly taught that the bad times for a woman's mental health are before her periods, after childbirth, and after the menopause (Priest and Crisp 1972; Priest and Steinert 1977), and that mental health is at its best *during* pregnancy. These are possibly oversimplified views. To a large extent the concept of freedom from mental illness *before* and excessive mental illness *after* delivery is based on the incidence of the most severe types of mental illness, i.e. psychoses. Doctors are taught that women rarely develop a psychosis during pregnancy but that they are very vulnerable during the weeks immediately following delivery. Any of the four main classes of psychosis can occur in the puerperium—organic, schizophrenic, depressive, or (rarely) manic. The acute organic brain syndrome (delirium) has become less common as bacterial infections have been controlled and the psychoses nowadays are usually one of the three remaining functional classes. As at other times of life depressive psychosis is commonest.

In addition depressive illness of a less disturbed type occurs in the weeks or months following delivery—depressive neurosis. Pitt (1966, 1967) has shown that over 10 per cent of women can be expected to develop such an illness. The patient with depressive neurosis does not suffer from delusions or hallucinations. There are various criteria for diagnosing an illness as neurotic (rather than within the normal everyday range of response of emotions) but Dr. Pitt's patients were suffering from an unusual degree of depression which was disabling and which made them ill for more than two weeks.

Depression may be part of frank mental illness, but women weep in other circumstances. The syndrome of 'post-partum blues' is an obvious example, occurring days after delivery and lasting only days. In addition *during* pregnancy women's emotions are notoriously labile and

7

Introduction

at the same time overt neurosis can occur.

Research has been carried out recently on the psychological sequelae of termination of pregnancy (Greer, Lal, Lewis, Belsey, and Beard 1976; Lask 1975; McCance, Olley, and Edward 1973; Priest 1972, 1978). In particular we can make some predictions about the likelihood of women developing depressive features of neurotic degree. Most of us know much less about post-abortion psychosis.

These are some of the categories of psychological disturbance that occur in relation to pregnancy. In this book we shall see whether our assumptions about them are correct, and what we can do about them when we come across them.

References

Lask, B. (1975). *Br. J. Psychiat.* **126**, 173.

McCance, C., Olley, P. C., and Edward, V. (1973). In *Experience with abortion: a case study of North-east Scotland* (ed. G. Horobin), pp. 245–300. Cambridge University Press.

Greer, H. S., Lal, S., Lewis, S. C., Belsey, D. M., and Beard, R. W. (1976). *Br. J. Psychiat.* **126**, 74.

Pitt, B. (1966). *A study of emotional disturbances associated with childbearing.* MD Thesis, University of London.

—— (1975). *Proc. roy. Soc. Med.* **68**, 223.

Priest, R. G. (1972). *Br. J. Psychiat.* **121**, 193.

—— (1978). In *Current themes in psychiatry* (ed. R. G. Gaind and B. Hudson), pp. 3–13, Macmillan, London.

—— and Crisp, A. H. (1972). In *Psychosomatic medicine in obstetrics and gynaecology* (ed. N. Morris), pp. 605–77. Karger, Basel.

—— and Steinert, J. (1977). *Insanity: a study of major psychiatric disorders.* Macdonald and Evans, Plymouth.

1

Some biological correlates of mental illness in relation to childbirth

M. SANDLER

According to traditional Hippocratic thought, melancholia derives from an excess of the humour, black bile, a suitable symbolic beginning for modern concepts of the biological origin of depressive illness. A number of somatic features of the disease—disturbance of sleep, appetite, bowel function, libido, and its frequent association with endocrine and other metabolic disorders—show that we are dealing with something more than a mere psychological upset. An obvious genetic component, together with the ability of certain stressful 'life events' to initiate acute episodes, must, again, give rise to a high index of suspicion. However, when we try to pinpoint the essential lesion, to search among these known biological correlates for clues to the aetiology of the condition, we immediately run into difficulties. It is against such an uncertain background that our attempts to scrutinize known biological correlates of mental illness in relation to childbirth must be viewed; they impose a further problematic dimension on a hazy and ambiguous canvas.

An anonymous leader writer in *The Lancet* (1978) has recently listed some of the difficulties which face the basic scientist in his study of depression. Any abnormal finding may reflect a primary difference at the core of the illness, a soocondary finding brought about by change in mood and activity or by drug treatment, or it may be an artefact associated with technique: 'Though there have been many apparent breakthroughs, time and again they have been like elephants' footprints in the mud, making a large initial impression but quickly fading into the background'. Thus, changes in electrolyte pattern (Coppen and Shaw 1963), in plasma cortisol concentrations (Gibbons and McHugh 1962) and in glucose tolerance (McCowan and Quastel 1931) have all been detected and none has yet emerged as being central to the biological upset of depressive illness.

Perhaps the leading hypothesis for the aetiology of this condition invokes a role for the monoamines. The monoamine hypothesis of depression was first adumbrated by Pare and Sandler (1959). It was formulated in greater detail and popularized by Schildkraut (1965) and, in essence, suggests that a deficiency of monoamine in the synaptic cleft may be responsible for attenuation of neurotransmission at this site. Thus, agents possessing the ability to step-up the concentration of monoamine in this site, monoamine oxidase inhibitors preventing destruction, or tricyclic antidepressants blocking re-uptake may well produce their therapeutic benefit by the local increase in monoamine they give rise to. The precise nature of the monoamine deficiency responsible for depressive illness, has remained somewhat shadowy. Schildkraut (1965) favoured noradrenaline as candidate; Lapin and Oxenkrug (1969) preferred 5-hydroxytryptamine; yet others (although their claims have been muted) have raised the possibility of dopamine as the deficient agent (Randrup, Munkvad, Fog, Gerlach, Molander, Kjellberg, and Scheel-Kruger 1975). It should be noted that these amines have in common the fact that all are present in discrete areas of the brain in relatively high concentration; thus, for a variety of reasons, they have been relatively easy to measure (Sandler 1972). However there is a spectrum of other monoamines, recently denominated 'trace amines' (Usdin and Sandler 1976; Baldessarini and Fischer 1978), not possessing the cerebral storage mechanisms largely responsible for the high local levels of the catecholamines and 5-hydroxytryptamine, but having a vigorous turnover in the body and, probably, in the brain where their distribution is discontinuous (Boulton 1974). All are substrates for the enzyme, monoamine oxidase, and this fact explains the careful re-examination this enzyme has undergone during the past decade (e.g. Costa and Sandler 1972; Wolstenholme and Knight 1976).

10

The simplistic hypothesis of Schildkraut (1965) has come under attack in recent years. In particular, Baldessarini (1975) has assembled a cogent series of arguments which clearly demonstrate its inadequacies. The tricyclic anti-depressant drugs may exert their effect by blocking the pre-synaptic re-uptake of monoamine in the synaptic cleft (Carlsson, Corrodi, Fuxe, and Höckfelt 1969a, b); however, one of the most telling recent arguments against the 'two-amine' hypothesis derives from the action of the antidepressant drugs, iprindole (Fann, Davis, Janowsky, Kaufmann, Griffith, and Oates, 1972) and mianserin (Leonard 1974) which are therapeutically effective yet have little or no action on monoamine re-uptake at presynaptic nerve endings. Perhaps for this reason more than any other, Kanof and Greengard (1978) have very lately turned their attention to a possible role for histamine and its receptor systems in the aetiology of depressive illness. They have pointed out that all tricyclic antidepressants have a significant interaction with histamine-sensitive adenylcyclase proportional to their antidepressant activity; this enzyme is likely to be intimately connected with the histamine receptor. Although their challenging idea obviously needs further evaluation, it does not take into account the antidepressant action of mono-amine oxidase inhibitors which, on the surface of it, have no obvious interaction with diamines such as histamine. It should be borne in mind, however, that the major meta-bolite of histamine in brain, methylhistamine (see Taylor 1975) has recently been shown to be an excellent substrate for monoamine oxidase B (Waldmeier, Feldtrauer, and Maitre 1977), one of the two major multiple forms of monoamine oxidase, according to latter-day theory (Johnston 1968).

The role of monoamine oxidase. Much of the diffi-culty in studying monoamine oxidase derives from the phys-icochemical nature of this enzyme which is insolubly bound to the outer membrane of the mitochondrion. Thus, although Johnston's subdivision into A and B forms has superseded an earlier classification based on electrophoretic mobility of the solubilized enzyme (Sandler and Youdim 1972), there is

11

still no absolute agreement that the apparent *in vitro* hetero-geneity is a true manifestation of an *in vivo* phenomenon. Although rat lung perfusion experiments after pretreatment with the selective MAO inhibitor, deprenyl (Roth and Gillis 1975; Bakhle and Youdim 1976), seem to point to the *in vivo* reality of the A-B classification, it seems to me equally likely that the apparent selectivity stems from some alternative pharmacological property of the drug employed. Other authors, too, have drawn attention to the possibility of the A-B classification being something of an over-simplification (Fowler, Callingham, Mantle, and Tipton 1978).

The subdivision into A and B forms of the enzyme was proposed to explain certain properties of the MAO inhibitor, clorgyline. The sigmoidal curve obtained from the action of different dilutions of the drug when tyramine was employed as substrate (Johnston 1968) was thus thought to derive from a selective inhibitory action against one component of the enzyme, termed MAO A. That portion of the enzyme resistant to the drug was termed MAO B. MAO A selectively oxidizes the 'classical' neurotransmitter monoamines, 5-hydroxy-tryptamine and noradrenaline. MAO B preferentially oxidizes phenylethylamine (Yang and Neff 1974), phenylethanol-amine (Edwards, D. J., personal communication) and methyl-histamine (Waldmeier *et al.* 1977). Tyramine and octopamine (Edwards and Venetti 1977) are substrates for both forms of the enzyme, a characteristic not without interest in assessing the significance of some new observations in this area de-scribed later in this paper.

The enzyme, monoamine oxidase, may be of particular importance within the female reproductive system and, indeed, there is some evidence to indicate that hormonal influences play a significant role in its regulation. Ten years ago, Southgate, Grant, Pollard, Pryse-Davies, and Sandler (1968) were able to show that there is a fairly sudden 'switching on' of monoamine oxidase activity in the human endometrium at about the 21st day of the menstrual cycle. This effect corresponds to peak plasma progesterone level. When progesterone is injected into rats, it brings about an

12

increase in MAO activity, particularly in the uterus (Collins, Pryse-Davies, Sandler, and Southgate 1970). The progesterone effect may well be significant at other sites in the body, particularly the brain (Holzbauer and Youdim 1973). It is tempting to speculate that such alterations in activity play some role in the depressive features which sometimes manifest in the premenstruum (although no very clear relationship can be defined between progesterone and depressive illness in the puerperium (see Chapter 8). Perhaps some overactivity of monoamine oxidase may consume disproportionately large amounts of amine which would otherwise be available to act as neurotransmitter in the synaptic cleft, in accordance with the monoamine hypothesis of depressive illness.

Very recently, my colleagues and I have updated these older observations and have been able to show that the progesterone effect is entirely confined to monoamine oxidase A, both in endometrium obtained late in the human menstrual cycle and in the progesterone-pretreated rat (Mazumder, R., Glover, V., and Sandler, M., in preparation).

The classification of monoamine oxidase into A and B forms was originally defined in terms of the selective inhibitor, clorgyline. At about the same time as this drug was synthesized, another compound, deprenyl, a selective monoamine oxidase B inhibitor, was being developed in Hungary. This drug has recently become of great therapeutic interest for it has been used in combination with L-dopa and a peripheral decarboxylase inhibitor as an adjuvant in the treatment of parkinsonism (Birkmayer, Riederer, Ambrozi, and Youdim 1977; Lees, Shaw, Kohout, Stern, Elsworth, Sandler, and Youdim 1977). The L-dopa derivative, dopamine, is preferentially oxidized in the human brain and platelet by monoamine oxidase B (Glover, Sandler, Owen, and Riley 1977), although in the gut mucosa (Squires 1972; Elsworth, Glover, Reynolds, Sandler, Lees, Phuapradit, Shaw, Stern, and Kumar 1978) and female reproductive tract (Mazumder, R., Glover, V., and Sandler, M., in preparation), it is a substrate for monoamine oxidase A. Deprenyl is of particular importance because its use, unlike that of other more classical monoamine oxidase inhibitors, does not put the patient at risk from the 'cheese effect' (Elsworth *et al.* 1978). Patients being treated with the more traditional inhibitors are likely to suffer profound hypertensive attacks when challenged with tyramine-containing compounds such as cheese (Marley and Blackwell 1970). Although Knoll (1976), the originator of this compound, has claimed that freedom from the 'cheese effect' derives mainly from the absence of mono-amine oxidase A inhibition, particularly in the gut wall, my colleagues and I have some recent evidence to show that this view is very much an oversimplification. Tyramine is thought to exert its hypertensive effect by liberating noradrenaline from its binding site and it seems likely that this releasing action may be interfered with in some other way (Sandler, M., Glover, V., and Ashford, A., to be published). This question is being actively investigated at the present time.

The role of trace amines. The role of tyramine in depressive illness, had it ever previously been considered at all, would have been relegated to that of adverse-reaction-producing agent during monoamine oxidase inhibitor therapy. Realizing that earlier investigations had largely concentrated on those monoamines which were stored in the brain, being consequently present in sufficient concentration to be assayed by relatively simple measuring procedures, my colleagues and I (Sandler, M., Goodwin, B. L., Ruthven, C. R. J., and Coppen, A., in preparation) decided to exploit recent methodological developments in this area and measure the excretory products of the 'trace amines'. Using gas chromatographic methods, supplemented where necessary by gas chromatographic-mass spectrometric procedures, we measured the urinary output of the major acidic metabolites of phenylethylamine (Goodwin, Ruthven, and Sandler 1975), o-, m- and p-tyramine, and p-octopamine (Goodwin, Ruthven, Fellows, and Sandler 1976). Significant decreases in output of p-hydroxyphenylacetic acid and p-hydroxymandelic acid, the major metabolites respectively of p-tyramine and p-octopamine were observed. It is of interest that these two compounds are linked in the biosynthetic chain, in that octopamine is formed from the β-hydroxylation of tyramine.

14

Although the excretion of phenylacetic acid, the major meta-
bolite of phenylethylamine, was not decreased in urine from
these patients—perhaps because any effect was disguised by
large amounts of these compounds deriving from diet or gut
flora (Sandler, Bonham Carter, Goodwin, and Ruthven
1976), subsequent work has shown that a significant decrease
of phenylacetic acid concentration was present in cerebrospinal fluid from affected subjects (Sandler, M., Goodwin,
B. L., Ruthven, C. R. J., and Coppen, A., in preparation).
Tyramine itself may be formed from the hydroxylation of
phenylethylamine, although this is still uncertain; the acidic
metabolites of tyramine and octopamine have not yet been
measured in cerebrospinal fluid from these depressed subjects, although such an investigation is in progress. It should
be mentioned in this context that parallel studies by Ghose,
Turner, and Coppen (1975) have revealed that depressed
patients manifest with an increase in pressor sensitivity to
intravenously administered tyramine compared with control
subjects. What may be of particular importance in this context is that this sensitivity does not disappear, even when the
patient's mental state has apparently returned to normal
(Coppen, A. and Ghose, K., personal communication). This
property has much in common, therefore, with the experiments described below, which have important overtones for
the possible prediction of puerperal depressive illness.

Tyramine conjugation deficit. Another abnormality
of tyramine metabolism which turned out to have significance in depressive illness first became apparent during an
investigation of patients with dietary migraine (Youdim,
Bonham Carter, Sandler, Hanington, and Wilkinson 1971;
Smith, Kellow, Mullen, and Hanington 1971). This group of
patients, whose headache was triggered off by certain items
of diet and most particularly by tyramine-containing foods
such as cheese (Hanington 1967), were observed to have an
apparent deficit in tyramine conjugation. When monoamines
in general are given orally, one pathway of metabolism which
is of minor significance for the degradation of the parenter-
ally administered substance assumes considerably greater

15

importance, sulphate conjugation. The proportion of amine metabolized by this route depends on its physicochemical nature. Thus, 60 per cent of *m*-octopamine is excreted as its sulphate conjugate (Hengstmann, Konen, Konen, Eichelbaum, and Dengler 1975) whilst *p*-tyramine is degraded to the extent of 10–15 per cent by this metabolic route (Sandler, Bonham Carter, Cuthbert, and Pare 1975) (Fig. 1).

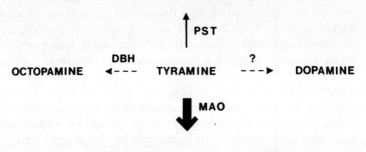

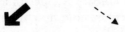

FIG. 1: Pathways of tyramine metabolism (from Sandler *et al.* 1975 by kind permission of the editor and publishers). Bold arrows show the major pathway. PST = phenolsulphotransferase; DBH = dopamine-β-hydroxylase; MAO = monoamine oxidase.

Because we (Sandler *et al.* 1975) thought, at that time, that the conjugation pathway represented a 'safety valve' mechanism, the impairment of which might cause danger to patients whose ability to metabolize monoamines by oxidative deamination was blocked by monoamine oxidase-inhibiting drugs, we investigated a series of subjects who were known to have had an adverse reaction whilst being so treated. In the course of this study, we discovered that *all* depressed patients under investigation, not only the affected

16

group, had an impaired conjugating ability. Very recently, we (Bonham Carter, Sandler, Goodwin, Sepping, and Bridges 1978a) tested a group of the most severely affected depressive subjects we could find, patients on whom all available physical and drug regimens had been tried without success. These medication-resistant patients were, therefore, considered suitable for modified leucotomy and the operation was duly performed. Before operation (Fig. 2), these subjects

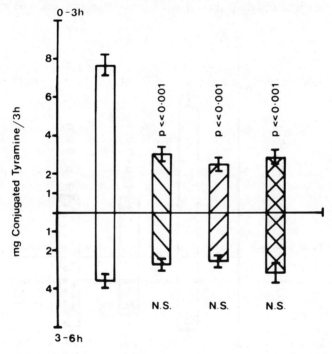

FIG. 2: Excretion of conjugated tyramine (mean ± SEM) after an oral tyramine load (100 mg) (from Bonham Carter *et al.* 1978a by kind permission of the editor and publishers). Key: ☐Controls. ◨Severely depressed patients (group 1), selected for modified leucotomy, pre-operatively. ◪Immediately post-operatively. ◈One year after operation. NS = not significantly different from control group.

showed a greater degree of impairment of conjugation than we had so far observed, more pronounced than that of the 'moderately depressed' group examined previously (Sandler *et al.* 1978). More remarkably, however, conjugated tyramine excretion in the first 3 h after tyramine ingestion remained low, not only post-operatively but in the follow-up group one year after operation. This was despite a dramatic improvement in the mental state of 6 out of 16 of them. The tyramine conjugation pattern was similarly impaired in responders and non-responders (Fig. 3). These findings seem to us to be extremely important, suggesting that even if the biochemical deficit is a pointer to the morbid predisposition, it is not immediately linked with the actual sequence of events

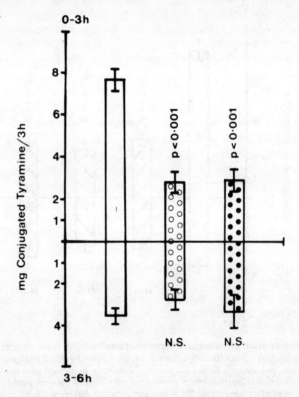

FIG. 3: Excretion of conjugated tyramine (mean ± SEM) after an oral tyramine load (100 mg) (from Bonham Carter *et al.* 1978a by kind permission of the editor and publishers). Key: □ Controls. ⊞ Severely depressed patients (group 1) assessed one year after modified leucotomy as 'recovered'. ◉ 'Unchanged'. NS = not significantly different from control group.

leading to a change in affect. It is of particular interest, within this context, that the enhanced pressor effect of tyramine in depressive illness (Ghose *et al.* 1975) also remains constant after recovery.

This present phase of investigation began with the observation that patients with a particular variety of migraine, that associated with tyramine sensitivity, was associated biochemically with a tyramine conjugation deficit. The recent observation of Ghose, Coppen, and Carroll (1977), that a sensitivity to the pressor action of tyramine is present in migraine, similar to the phenomenon they demonstrated in depression (Ghose *et al.* 1975), is thus particularly noteworthy. Although accounts have been largely anecdotal, it should be noted that some authors have drawn attention to a degree of clinical overlap between the two conditions (e.g. Couch, Ziegler, and Hassanein 1975) and, indeed, certain patients with intractable migraine may respond to drugs usually administered for depressive illness—monoamine oxidase inhibitors (Anthony and Lance 1969), tricyclic antidepressants (Gomersall and Stuart 1973), lithium (Ekbom 1974)—when standard therapeutic regimens have failed. Thus, exaggerated tyramine pressor sensitivity and impaired tyramine conjugation are probably common manifestations of the state of vulnerability shared by the two illnesses. This concept would visualize the florid disease making its appearance only after an appropriate triggering event, presumably involving a different mechanism for each clinical condition.

The classification of depressive illness is difficult and controversial (Kendell 1976). To identify the physical counterparts of the disease, whatever their mechanism of origin, may well be helpful diagnostically. We may, for example, be able to identify the proportion of patients whose alcoholism has a depressive component (Seixas 1977). It is within the context of the present discussion that the ability of the oral tyramine test to identify a predisposition to depressive illness may prove its true worth. A sharp rise in the incidence of depressive episodes in the months following childbirth is well documented (Pitt 1975; Kendell, Wainwright, Hailey, and Shannon 1976). Preliminary information deriving from a

19

recent survey here at Queen Charlotte's Hospital would confirm this high incidence—application of the Zung self-rating depression scale (Zung 1965) to women returning to hospital for check-up six weeks after giving birth revealed a rate of seven per cent falling into the depressive category (unpublished), a figure agreeing fairly well with other estimates. It is now generally accepted that maternal illness of this type may, to a varying extent, be reflected in a corresponding infant morbidity (see Chapter 12) ranging from minor disorders such as fretfulness and feeding difficulties to problems as grave as the battered baby syndrome (Smith 1973). Thus, if the potentially depressive mother could be identified in advance by a predictive test such as the oral tyramine test, prompt medical and social care could do much to improve her quality of life and avert any deleterious effect on her child. We have now embarked upon a large-scale prospective study at Queen Charlotte's Hospital to test the validity of this concept, involving the combined efforts of obstetricians, psychiatrists, psychologists, nursing staff, and social workers, with appropriate laboratory back-up.

There remains one important outstanding question, the nature of the apparent tyramine conjugation defect. Preliminary work has already indicated that a sulphate deficit is unlikely to be responsible (Bonham Carter, Sandler, Sepping, and Bridges 1978b), as claimed by another team (Smith and Mitchell 1974). However, as both our groups have employed inorganic sulphate supplements to test this concept, we are repeating the experiments after the administration of cysteine which is well absorbed from the gastrointestinal tract, unlike the sulphate ion. We (Sandler *et al.* 1975) have also speculated previously about the deficit deriving from a possible increase in monoamine oxidase activity so that a relatively small amount of tyramine would be available for sulphate conjugation. However we have not been able to demonstrate any convincing increase in urinary output of *p*-hydroxyphenylacetic acid, the major metabolite of tyramine (Bonham Carter *et al.* 1978a) (Fig. 1), whilst patients in our medication-resistant group of patients were resistant to monoamine oxidase inhibitor therapy in addition to other drugs.

Although we (Sandler *et al.* 1975) originally thought that we were able to rule out an actual decreased activity of the conjugating enzyme, which is largely located in the gut wall (Morgan, Ruthven, and Sandler 1969), using an indirect approach, certain flaws in our experimental design have since become apparent so that this possibility needs to be ruled out by direct observation, involving gut biopsy. The unitary hypothesis we tend to favour above all others, however, is that involving some impedance of membrane transport throughout the body, caused by a defect in an as yet unknown mechanism. This might well account for a number of observations scattered through the literature which by themselves are difficult to explain (Bonham Carter *et al.* 1978a). Because such a general impedance might affect the initial mixing phase of antipyrine, a drug widely used for the evaluation of body water space, we have recently tried to test the hypothesis by administering this drug to a number of depressive and control subjects; we failed to find any difference between them (Bonham Carter, Sandler, Bridges, and Davies, to be published). However, it should be remembered that apart from a few islands of detailed information, our knowledge of biological transport systems is in its infancy (Christensen 1975). My colleagues and I consider that the investigation of membrane structure and transport function in patients with depressive illness might be a fruitful future avenue of research. The supplementary question, involving possible additional or parallel changes in membrane transport in pregnancy and the puerperium, has hardly yet been formulated. The concept might well deserve careful evaluation in the future.

References

Anthony, M. and Lance, J. W. (1969). *Arch. Neurol.* 21, 263.

Bakhle, Y. S. and Youdim, M. B. H. (1976). *Br. J. Pharmac.* 56, 125.

Baldessarini, R. J. (1975). *Arch. gen. Psychiat.* 32, 1087.

—— and Fischer, J. E. (1978). *Biochem. Pharmac.* 27, 621.

Birkmayer, W., Riederer, P., Ambrozi, L., and Youdim, M. B. H. (1977). *Lancet* i, 439.

21

Some biological correlates of mental

Bonham Carter, S., Sandler, M., Goodwin, B. L., Sepping, P., and Bridges, P. K. (1978a). *Br. J. Psychiat.* 132, 125.

— — — Sepping, P., and Bridges, P. K. (1978b). *Br. J. clin. Pharmac.* 5, 269.

Boulton, A. A. (1974). *Lancet* ii, 52.

Carlsson, A., Corrodi, H., Fuxe, K., and Hökfelt, T. (1969a). *Eur. J. Pharmac.* 5, 357.

— — — — — (1969b). *Eur. J. Pharmac.* 5, 367.

Christensen, H. N. (1975). *Biological transport* (2nd edn.). Benjamine Reading, Massachusetts.

Collins, G. G. S., Pryse-Davies, J., Sandler, M., and Southgate, J. (1970). *Nature* 226, 642.

Coppen, A. and Shaw, D. M. (1963). *Br. med. J.* ii, 1439.

Costa, E. and Sandler, M. (eds.) (1972). *Monoamine oxidases—new vistas*. Raven, New York.

Couch, J. R., Ziegler, D. J., and Hassanein, R. (1975). *Headache* 15, 41.

Edwards, D. J. and Venetti, M. C. (1977). *Neurosci. Abstr.* 3, 313.

Ekbom, K. (1974). *Opusc. Med.* 19, 148.

Elsworth, J. D., Glover, V., Reynolds, G. P., Sandler, M., Lees, A. J., Phuapradit, P., Shaw, K. M., Stern, G. M., and Kumar, P. (1978). *Psychopharmacology* 57, 33.

Fann, W. E., Davis, J. M., Janowsky, D. S., Kaufmann, J. S., Griffith, J. D., and Oates, J. A. (1972). *Arch. gen. Psychiat.* 26, 158.

Fowler, C. J., Callingham, B. A., Mantle, T. J., and Tipton, K. F. (1978). *Biochem. Pharmac.* 27, 97.

Ghose, K., Turner, P., and Coppen, A. (1975). *Lancet* i, 1317.

— — Coppen, A., and Carroll, D. (1977). *Br. med. J.* i, 1191.

Gibbons, J. L. and McHugh, P. R. (1962). *J. psychiat. Res.* 1, 162.

Glover, V., Sandler, M., Owen, F., and Riley, G. J. (1977). *Nature* 265, 80.

Gomersall, J. D. and Stuart, A. (1973). *J. Neurol. Neurosurg. Psychiat.* 36, 684.

Goodwin, B. L., Ruthven, C. R. J., and Sandler, M. (1975). *Clin. chim. Acta* 62, 443.

— — — Fellows, L. E., and Sandler, M. (1976). *Clin. chim. Acta* 73, 191.

Hanington, E. (1967). *Br. med. J.* ii, 550.

Hengstmann, J. A., Konen, W., Konen, C., Eichelbaum, M., and Dengler, H. J. (1975). *Eur. J. clin. Pharmac.* 8, 33.

Holzbauer, M. and Youdim, M. B. H. (1973). *Br. J. Pharmac.* 48, 600.

Johnston, J. P. (1968). *Biochem. Pharmac.* 17, 1285.

Kanof, P. D. and Greengard, P. (1978). *Nature* 272, 329.

Kendell, R. E. (1976). *Br. J. Psychiat.* 129, 15.

— — Wainwright, S., Hailey, A., and Shannon, B. (1976). *Psychol. Med.* 6, 297.

Knoll, J. (1976), In *Monoamine oxidase and its inhibition* (ed. G. E. W.

22

Wolstenholme and J. Knight), p. 135. Elsevier-Excerpta Medica-North Holland, Amsterdam.

The Lancet (1978) i, 422.

Lapin, I. P. and Oxenkrug, G. F. (1969). *Lancet* i, 132.

Lees, A. J., Shaw, K. M., Kohout, L. J., Stern, G. M., Elsworth, J. D., Sandler, M., and Youdim, M. B. H. (1977). *Lancet* ii, 791.

Leonard, B. E. (1974). *Psychopharmacologia* 36, 221.

McCowan, P. K. and Quastel, J. H. (1931). *J. ment. Sci.* 77, 525.

Marley, E. and Blackwell, B. (1970). *Advan. Pharmac. Chemother.* 8, 196.

Morgan, C. D., Ruthven, C. R. J., and Sandler, M. (1969). *Clin. chim. Acta* 26, 381.

Pare, C. M. B. and Sandler, M. (1959). *J. Neurol. Neurosurg. Psuchiat.* 22, 247.

Pitt, B. (1975). *Br. J. Psychiat.* Spec. No. 9, 409.

Randrup, A., Munkvad, I., Fog, R., Gerlach, J., Molander, L., Kjellberg, B., and Scheel-Kruger, J. (1975). In *Current developments in psychopharmacology* (ed. W. B. Essman and L. Valzelli), Vol. 2, p. 205. Spectrum, New York.

Roth, J. A. and Gillis, C. N. (1975). *J. Pharmac. exp. Ther.* 94, 537.

Sandler, M. (1972). *Proc. roy. Soc. Med.* 65, 584.

—— and Youdim, M. B. H. (1972). *Pharmac. Rev.* 24, 331.

—— Bonham Carter S., Cuthbert, M. F., and Pare, C. M. B. (1975). *Lancet* i, 1045.

—— — Goodwin, B. L., and Ruthven, C. R. J. (1976). In *Trace amines and the brain* (ed. E. Usdin and M. Sandler), p. 233. Dekker, New York.

Schildkraut, J. J. (1965). *Am. J. Psychiat.* 122, 509.

Seixas, F. (ed.) (1977). *Currents in alcoholism*, Vol. 2. Psychiatric, psychological, social, and epidemiological studies. Grune and Stratton, New York.

Smith, I., Kellow, A. H., Mullen, P. E., and Hanington, E. (1971). *Nature*, 230, 246.

—— and Mitchell, P. D. (1974). *Biochem. J.* 142, 189.

Smith, S. M (1973). *The battered child syndrome*. Butterworth, London.

Southgate, J., Grant, E. C., Pollard, W., Pryse-Davies, J., and Sandler, M. (1968). *Biochem. Pharmac.* 17, 721.

Squires, R. F. (1972). In *Monoamine oxidases—new vistas* (ed. E. Costa and M. Sandler), p. 355. Raven, New York.

Taylor, K. M. (1975). In *Handbook of psychopharmacology* (ed. L. L. Iversen, S. D. Iversen, and S. H. Snyder), Vol. 3, p. 327. Plenum, New York.

Usdin, E. and Sandler, M. (eds.) (1976). *Trace amines and the brain*. Dekker, New York.

Waldmeier, P. C., Feldtrauer, J.-J., and Maitre, L. (1977). *J. Neurochem.* 29, 785.

Wolstenholme, G. E. W. and Knight, J. (eds.) (1976). *Monoamine oxidase and its inhibition.* Elsevier-Excerpta Medica-North Holland, Amsterdam.

Yang, H.-Y. T. and Neff, N. H. (1974). *J. Pharmac. exp. Ther.* **189**, 733.

Youdim, M. B. H., Bonham Carter, S., Sandler, M., Hanington, E., and Wilkinson, M. (1971). *Nature* **230**, 127.

Zung, W. W. K. (1965). *Arch. gen. Psychiat.* **12**, 63.

2

Postnatal depression and tryptophan metabolism

A. COPPEN, G. STEIN, and K. WOOD

The role of 5-hydroxytryptamine (5-HT) in the affective disorders has been the subject of much research and was originally suggested by the elucidation of some of the mechanisms of action of antidepressant drugs. The tricyclic antidepressant drugs inhibit the re-uptake of released amines and the monoamine oxidase (MAO) inhibitors reduce the intracellular deamination of 5-HT. Investigations of disturbances of 5-HT metabolism in depressive illness have included measurements of 5-HT levels in the brains of depressive suicides (Bourne, Bunney, Colburn, Davis, Davis, Shaw, and Coppen 1968) and the concentration of the metabolite of 5-HT, 5-hydroxyindoleacetic acid (5-HIAA) in the cerebrospinal fluid of depressive patients (van Praag, Korf, and Puite 1970; Coppen, Prange, Whybrow, and Noguera 1972). The results of these investigations and their interpretation have been conflicting but there is increasing evidence of a disturbance of 5-HT metabolism in depressive illness. 5-HT in the brain is derived from tryptophan and the rate-limiting-enzyme (tryptophan 5-hydroxylase) in its synthesis is not saturated with substrate (Green and Grahame-Smith 1975). The concentration of tryptophan in the brain and its availability from the plasma is of great importance. Tryptophan, unlike other amino acids, is bound to plasma proteins (McMenamy and Oncley 1958). Therefore, the unbound or free fraction in plasma is important in determining tryptophan concentration in the brain (Tagliamonte, Tagliamonte, Perez-Cruet, Stern, and Gessa 1971). Another factor which may influence levels of brain tryptophan is the concentration of other amino acids (leucine, isoleucine, valine, tyrosine, and

25

phenylalanine) which compete with tryptophan for transport into the brain (Fernstrom and Wurtman 1972). It has been suggested, however, that total plasma tryptophan is the relevant index for predicting brain tryptophan concentration (Fernstrom, Hirsch, and Faller 1976).

In an investigation to determine the concentration of tryptophan in the plasma of depressed patients we reported a reduced concentration of free tryptophan in the plasma of depressed patients (Table 2.1) (Coppen, Eccleston, and Peet 1973a). These initial findings have been confirmed by some workers (Aylward 1973; Kishimoto and Hama 1976) but not by others (Niskanen, Huttunen, Tamminen, and Jaaskelainen 1976). The combination of monoamine oxidase inhibitors and tryptophan (Coppen, Shaw, and Farrell 1963) and tricyclic antidepressants and tryptophan (Walinder, Skott, Nagy, Carlsson, and Roos 1975) have clearly been shown to be effective treatments for depression.

In contrast to the severe disturbances of mood observed in endogenous depression, mild disturbances of mood occur in 50–70 per cent of women during the post-partum period (Yalom, Lunde, and Moos 1968). Three to four days after the birth of their child some women begin to cry for no apparent reason. The crying may be intense and prolonged and may often, but not always, be associated with a depressed mood. These mood changes, therefore, prompted us to examine the relationship between levels of tryptophan in the plasma of women during the puerperium and their affective state (Stein, Milton, Bebbington, Wood, and Coppen 1976). These concentrations have been compared to those found in normal female controls.

A pilot study showed that mood disturbances were most severe on the sixth day post-partum, and hence we selected the sixth day for the estimation of plasma tryptophan levels. Eighteen women in a post-natal ward were interviewed 24h after the birth of their child and invited to participate in the investigation. They rated themselved daily during their subsequent seven or eight days in hospital on a series of scales for five symptoms:

Tearfulness = 0 (no tears) to 4 (cried for more than 30 min);
Depression = 0 (no depression) to 4 (very depressed);
Anxiety = 0 (normal anxiety) to 4 (desperately anxious);
Appetite = 0 (normal appetite) to 4 (complete loss of appetite);
Insomnia = 0 (good night's sleep) to 4 (very disturbed sleep).

An average daily score for each symptom for every patient was calculated, and the sum of the average, daily scores for each symptom provided an average 'total affective score'. Thus, the maximum possible average daily score per symptom was 4 and the maximum daily 'total affective score' was 20, which enabled us to rank the patients in order of increasing affective disturbance.

The patients fasted from 10 p.m. on the previous night and took no medication. They awoke at 5.30 a.m. to feed their babies and had a cup of tea and then fasted until 9 a.m. when 30 ml of venous blood were collected and placed in heparinized bottles. The plasma was separated by centrifuging and total and free plasma tryptophan concentrations were estimated (Eccleston 1973). The levels found in a group of normal controls are shown for comparison. Table 2.2 shows groups of post-partum patients in order of increasing affective disturbance together with their tryptophan levels.

Patients who appeared clinically to have severe depression (ranks 15–18) had free plasma tryptophan concentrations similar to those found in depressive illness. Only one of the remaining patients (rank 7) had a low free tryptophan level (4·6 μmol/l) and she appeared to be hypomanic. Free plasma tryptophan correlated significantly with depression ($r = -0·60; p < 0·01$) and also with the total affective score ($r = -0·49; p < 0·05$). The other symptoms showed similar trends but the correlations did not reach statistical significance. Total plasma tryptophan did not correlate with any of the clinical data but was 33·5 per cent higher than in the controls. In order to obtain a clear picture of changes in total and free plasma tryptophan we studied the concentrations of plasma tryptophan in nineteen women in the 35th or 36th week of pregnancy (Coppen, Stein, and Wood 1977a). The concentration of plasma free tryptophan in the

Table 2.1. *Mean plasma tryptophan concentrations in female depressive patients and controls*

	N	Mean age (years)	Free tryptophan (μmol l^{-1})	Total tryptophan (μmol l^{-1})
Control subjects	51	47·7 ± 0·8	6·71 ± 0·25	58·8 ± 1·47
Depressed patients	50	55·1 ± 1·9	4·07* ± 0·20	59·8 ± 1·47

All figures are expressed ± S.E.
*Depressed patients significantly less ($p < 0.001$) than controls.

Table 2.2. *Mean plasma tryptophan concentration in the post-partum patients ranked in order of increasing severity of affective disturbances*

	N	Rank no.	Mean total affective score	Mean age (years)	Free plasma tryptophan (μmol l^{-1})	Total plasma tryptophan (μmol l^{-1})
Post-partum patients	18	1–5	0·75 ± 0·10	27·6 ± 2·7	7·00 ± 0·93	82·3 ± 4·1
		6–10	1·79 ± 0·09	29·6 ± 3·0	6·51 ± 0·54	86·7 ± 4·2
		11–14	2·31 ± 0·14	25·8 ± 0·6	6·76 ± 0·59	89·1 ± 5·5
		15–18	5·10 ± 0·90	25·0 ± 1·7	4·36 ± 0·49	80·8 ± 5·3
Normal female controls	16			25·6 ± 0·8	5·93* ± 0·34	56·3** ± 1·6

All figures are expressed ± S.E.
*Difference from patient ranks 15–18, $p < 0.05$.
**Difference from patient ranks 1–18, $p < 0.001$.

Table 2.3. *Mean plasma tryptophan levels in pre-partum women, post-partum women, and a group of normal female controls*

	N	Mean age (years)	Free plasma tryptophan (μmol l^{-1})	Total plasma tryptophan (μmol l^{-1})
Pre-partum	19	26·7 ± 1·3	5·06* ± 0·34	42·0** ± 0·9
Post-partum	18	27·4 ± 1·2	6·22 ± 0·39	84·7*** ± 2·3
Normal female controls	16	25·6 ± 0·8	5·93 ± 0·34	56·3** ± 1·6

All figures are expressed ± S.E.
*Significantly lower than post-partum group, $p < 0.05$.
**Significantly different from one another, $p < 0.001$.

pre-partum group (Table 2.3) was lower but not significantly so than in the normal controls but was significantly lower ($p < 0.05$) than in the post-partum group which contained patients some of whom suffered from affective disturbance. The levels of total tryptophan in the plasma of the pre-partum group were significantly lower ($p < 0.001$) than normal controls and significantly lower than the post-partum group ($p < 0.001$).

The results of our initial study show a significant correlation between severity of affective disturbances and free plasma tryptophan levels. A similar relationship has recently been detected by Handley, Dunn, Baker, Cockshott, and Gould (1977). Hence, mood changes in the post-partum period may be mediated by changes in brain 5-HT and free plasma tryptophan, as may be the case with depressive illness. Decreased 5-HT turnover has been reported in hypomania, and the one patient in our series who appeared to be hypomanic had a low free plasma tryptophan level.

The reduced concentration of total tryptophan in the plasma of pre-partum women compared with controls and post-partum patients may be due to the increases in blood and plasma volume that occur during pregnancy. Increases of up to approximately 50 per cent of the normal plasma volume are observed between the 68th and 5th day before childbirth, i.e. at the time when these investigations were carried out. The total amount of tryptophan in the blood may be increased compared with the non-pregnant state although the actual concentration of tryptophan may be decreased. The total amount of tryptophan in the maternal circulation may therefore be adequate to meet the demands of the mother and foetus. Abnormal levels of free tryptophan associated with affective disturbance may be due in part to the considerable changes in plasma volume and also to the considerable hormonal changes occurring after childbirth which influence tryptophan binding.

Affective disorders occur commonly for the first time in the fourth decade of life. The menopause (when there are decreases in the level of circulating oestrogens) has been implicated as a possible contributory factor in the onset of the illness. To investigate the effect of the menopause and age on total and free plasma tryptophan we examined the concentrations of plasma tryptophan in normal subjects (Coppen and Wood 1978). The mean age of the menopause was based on an epidemiological study (Jaszmann 1976) and was found to be 51·4 years with a standard deviation of 3·8 years. The subjects were then divided into 3 age groups, i.e., ≤ 46 years (premenopausal), 47-55 years (perimenopausal) and ≥ 56 years (postmenopausal). The concentration of plasma free tryptophan obtained from normal subjects is shown in Table 2.4. The perimenopausal group had a significantly lower free plasma tryptophan concentration than the pre- and post-menopausal group. No significant difference in total tryptophan concentration was detected within any of the groups in the normal control subjects. This reduced level of free tryptophan during the menopause may be due in part to the decrease in oestrogens which occurs during the menopause and could be a contributory factor to the mood changes commonly observed at this time.

The effects of oestrogens on plasma tryptophan levels have been investigated in a double-blind cross-over trial (Coppen, Rao, Ghose, and Wood 1978). Female patients attending a prophylactic lithium clinic were studied. These patients had mild residual affective symptoms but were not seriously disturbed. Each patient was randomly assigned to receive initially either active oestrogen or placebo oestrogen. The patients were kept on an active regime when they received 1·25 mg conjugated oestrogens (Premarin, Ayerst Laboratories Ltd., Camberley, Surrey, U.K.), once daily for 12 weeks. Before treatment commenced, and at the end of placebo and active treatment, total and free tryptophan were estimated at the same time as affective morbidity was measured (Beck, Ward, Mendelson, Mock, and Erbaugh 1961; Coppen, Peet, Bailey, Noguera, Burns, Swani, Maggs, and Gardner 1973b). The results of these measurements are presented in Table 2.5.

No significant difference in depressive symptoms could be found between the 2 treatment regimens. There was a significant ($p < 0.02$) increase in level of free tryptophan when

Table 2.4. *Relationship between total and free plasma tryptophan and age in a group of normal controls*

	Age group	N	Total plasma tryptophan (μmol l^{-1})	Free plasma tryptophan (μmol l^{-1})
Control subjects	$\leqslant 46$	20	$58 \cdot 2 \pm 2 \cdot 3$	$7 \cdot 06 \pm 0 \cdot 49$
	$47-55$	20	$58 \cdot 7 \pm 1 \cdot 8$	$6 \cdot 18* \pm 0 \cdot 25$
	$\geqslant 56$	11	$59 \cdot 7 \pm 2 \cdot 6$	$7 \cdot 25 \pm 0 \cdot 59$

All figures expressed as means ± S.E.
*Significantly different from control pre- and post-menopausal group, $p < 0 \cdot 05$.

Table 2.5. *Mean total and free plasma tryptophan levels in a group of female patients on oestrogen (active and placebo) treatment*

	N	On placebo	On oestrogen
Total tryptophan (μmol l^{-1})	9	$59 \cdot 8 \pm 2 \cdot 94$	$65 \cdot 2 \pm 2 \cdot 94$
Free tryptophan (μmol l^{-1})	9	$3 \cdot 24 \pm 0 \cdot 34$	$5 \cdot 10* \pm 0 \cdot 34$
Affective morbidity	9	$0 \cdot 32 \pm 0 \cdot 09$	$0 \cdot 35 \pm 0 \cdot 13$
Beck IMD	9	$9 \cdot 7 \pm 2 \cdot 5$	$8 \cdot 7 \pm 2 \cdot 7$

All figures are expressed ± S.E.
*Active vs. placebo, $p < 0 \cdot 02$.

the patients were on the active oestrogen treatment compared with placebo group. This effect is probably a direct one since *in vitro* oestrogens displace tryptophan from plasma protein binding sites (Aylward 1973). The reason for the lack of therapeutic effect may be that lithium, perhaps exerting its action by increasing brain tryptophan or releasing 5-HT, obscured any therapeutic effect of oestrogen. The mild affective morbidity of the patients was not changed significantly. The decrease in the free tryptophan concentration observed at the perimenopausal stage may therefore be related to the decrease in circulating oestrogens which occurs at the same time. Although oestrogens did not alleviate the mild residual affective symptoms in a group of female depressed patients attending a prophylactic lithium clinic, they have a significant effect in increasing concentrations of plasma free tryptophan. Elsewhere, a report on the action of oestrone sulphate on post-hysterectomized women suggests that oestrogens may reduce affective morbidity (Coppen, Bishop, and Beard 1977b).

It is possible, therefore, that the hormonal fluctuations induced by pregnancy and childbirth in plasma free tryptophan concentrations, may account for some of the psychiatric disturbances associated with both the post-partum period and the menopause.

We wish to thank Mr. Diggory, Mr. Macgrath, Mr. Fairburn, and Mr. Gordon for allowing us to study the patients under their care and gratefully acknowledge the help of Sisters Clark, Wilton, and Stuart-Menteth. We thank Mrs. J. Harwood and Miss M. Bishop for technical assistance. We thank Mr. J. E. Bailey for statistical analysis of the data.

References

Aylward, M. (1973). *I.R.C.S. med. Sci. J.* 1, 30.

Beck, A. T., Ward, C. M., Mendelson, M., Mock, J., and Erbaugh, J. (1961). *Arch. gen. Psychiat.* 4, 561.

Bourne, H. R., Bunney, W. E., Colburn, R. W., Davis, J. M., Davis, N. J., Shaw, D. M., and Coppen, A. J. (1968). *Lancet* ii, 805.

Coppen, A., Shaw, D. M., and Farrell, J. P. (1963). *Lancet* i, 79.

—— Prange, A. J., Whybrow, P., and Noguera, R. (1972). *Arch. gen. Psychiat.* 26, 474.

—— Eccleston, E. G., and Peet, M. (1973a). *Lancet* ii, 60.

—— Peet, M., Bailey, J., Noguera, R. Burns, B. M., Swani, M. S., Maggs, R., and Gardner, R. (1973b). *Psychiat. Neurol. Neurochir.* 76, 501.

—— and Wood, K. (1978). *Psychol. Med.* 8, 49.

—— Stein, G., and Wood, K. (1977a). *Res. Commun. Psychol. Psychiat. Behav.* 2, 235.

—— Bishop, M., and Beard, R. J. (1977b). *Curr. med. Res. Opinion* 4, 29.

—— Rao, V. A. R., Ghose, K., and Wood, K. (1978). *Int. J. Pharmacopsychiat.*, in press.

Eccleston, E. G. (1973). *Clin. chim. Acta* 48, 269.

Fernstrom, J. D. and Wurtman, R. J. (1972). *Science* 178, 414.

—— Hirsch, M. J., and Faller, D. V. (1976). *Biochem. J.* 160, 589.

Green, A. R. And Grahame-Smith, D. G. (1975). In *Handbook of psychopharmacology* (ed. L. L. Iversen, S. B. Iversen, and S. H. Snyder), vol. 3, p. 169. Plenum Press, New York.

Handley, S. L., Dunn, T. L., Baker, J. M., Cockshott, C., and Gould, S. (1977). *Br. med. J.* ii, 18.

Jaszmann, L. L. B. (1976). In *The Management of the menopause and post-menopausal years* (ed. S. Campbell), p. 11. MTP Press, Lancaster.

Kishimoto, M. and Hama, Y. (1976). *Yokohama med. Bull.* 27, 89.

McMenamy, R. H. and Oncley, J. L. (1958). *J. biol. Chem.* 233, 1436.

Niskanen, P., Huttunen, M., Tamminen, T., and Jaaskelainen, J. (1976). *Br. J. Psychiat.* 128, 67.

Stein, G., Milton, F., Bebbington, P., Wood, K., and Coppen, A. (1976). *Br. med. J.* ii, 457.

Tagliamonte, A., Tagliamonte, P., Perez-Cruet, J., Stern, S., and Gessa, G. L. (1971). *J. Pharmac. exp. Ther.* 177, 475.

Van Praag, H. M., Korf, J., and Puite, J. (1970). *Nature* 225, 1259.

Wålinder, J., Skott, A., Nagy, A., Carlssen, A., and Roos, B.-E. (1975). *Lancet* i, 984.

Yalom, I. D., Lunde, D. T., and Moos, R. M. (1968). *Arch. gen Psychiat.* 18, 16.

3
Mental illness and its obstetric management

C. H. NAYLOR

Occasionally we obstetricians need to remind ourselves about the fundamental personal needs, desires, and hopes of our pregnant patients. Apart from their pregnancy they are just like others, dependent on love, companionship, the approval of others, and physical and emotional comfort and security. How, for instance, are the fundamental needs satisfied in the case of a young primigravida with pre-eclampsia at 34 weeks gestation who has to face an indeterminate in-patient stay of up to four weeks? During this time her baby's life is at risk from anoxia or asphyxia or, if labour is induced, from respiratory distress and prematurity. Her own physical well-being is threatened by acute hypertension, which can lead to cerebral oedema, loss of consciousness, fits, and eclampsia. This condition carries a maternal mortality of 5 per cent. Pre-eclampsia has been suggested as a predisposing factor to mental illness. Currently I am having great difficulty in making a differential diagnosis between severe mental illness and brain damage in a patient who recently developed eclampsia.

When the achievement of a goal (perhaps in the case of pregnancy, the delivery of a healthy baby) is blocked, denied, or threatened, and an individual's personal integrity is threatened, emotions are aroused mobilizing energy for action. The intensity of the reaction varies. There may be a minor response, annoyance, or there may be a major response with intense anger, hatred, or fear. The outcome depends on three factors—the personal significance of the situation, the constitutional make-up of the patient, and her past experience in handling the day-to-day problems of life. In most

35

instances there is satisfactory resolution.

But action may be blocked, behaviour not tolerated; there may be social censorship, or there may be a moral dilemma, and there may be a threat to the individual's security. The aroused energy persists and increases in intensity as the patient fails to cope with the current problem. There is usually powerful, unspent, emotional energy and this causes alterations in the patient's physiological and psychological capacity to adapt. It is possible to identify and evaluate these failures clinically. In psychological failure there is first a disturbance of attitude and feeling and this may lead to depression, hypomania or mania. There are associated subjective symptoms of anxiety, fear, irritability, tension, and mood changes. There will be a change in patterns of sleep, appetite, work, and recreation. Often there is insomnia at night and lassitude during the day. The patient becomes less tolerant and complains of her inability to carry on.

During gestation, there are profound physiological changes in the endocrine system, the autonomic nervous system, and in circulating fluid, and an increase in cardiac output. There is a change in body shape; there may be vomiting, diarrhoea, frequency of micturition, and minor symptoms relating to almost every system in the body. Pregnancy is unique. Psychologically, there is great emotional energy requiring adaptation rather than action.

The physiological changes increase as pregnancy progresses and the patient has to come to terms and accept a new responsibility that will be spread over many years. A patient's attitude to pregnancy will depend on a number of factors— her past experience of illness and admission to hospital, her degree of maturity, stability, and security, and the attitude and behaviour of the husband and other members of her family, the in-laws, and perhaps her current social and economic status. An obstetrician must assess the patient's emotional and psychosexual growth and development. Anatomical and physiological growth and development of the female genital tract and secondary sexual characteristics progress to maturity along well-defined inherited tracks, in marked contrast with emotional and psychosexual growth and development which are not determined by similar inherited tendencies. There is no assurance that full emotional and psychosexual maturity will ever be achieved. The attitude and behaviour of her parents and environmental, social, cultural, and economic factors all influence development. What determines the achievement of adult femininity? There must be full acceptance of the feminine role with self-love and self-approval, with acceptance of the female body as basically healthy and the physiological functions, especially those of menstruation, as normal. There should be acceptance of sexual need and urges as normal, healthy, emotional and physical manifestations of male and female. Parental example should lead to acceptance of and eager anticipation of marriage, pregnancy, and motherhood as natural, normal, and desirable events for the future.

Emotional resources can be assessed in three areas—first, acceptance of the pregnancy and child; second, the patient's degree of stability and maturity; and, third, the assessment of factors in her environment. A deficiency of one can be compensated by strength in another. If she has a positive attitude to pregnancy and anticipates the child, the prognosis is good. If the pregnancy has been planned, this is a favourable feature, although in a study of patients attending an outpatient department in West London, 40 per cent of the patients admitted that the pregnancy was unplanned. There should be pride and self-identity as a mother or a mother-to-be and a determination to remain healthy and normal with minimization of discomfort from the anatomical and physiological changes of pregnancy. In assessing the patient's degree of emotional stability and maturity, one must consider her acceptance of the feminine role with no unreasonable fears about herself and her baby. Family training and good health care is a favourable sign. Has she the capacity to establish friendships among the nurses and obstetricians and to accept instructions from them regarding her health care? Does she have a history of an ability to adapt to new life situations? Has she a favourable educational work record, and has she good self-identification as a wife in a marriage which is reasonably stable? In considering the stability of her environment, one must consider the attitude of her husband. Was he keen on the pregnancy? Does he anticipate the child? Has he pride in self-identity as a father or father-to-be? Does he accept the pregnancy as being normal? Has he confidence in midwives and doctors? Has he a favourable educational and work record? Has he the ability to provide a home environment of love and security? An ability to help resolve temporary feelings of insecurity, fears and mood changes with the physical discomforts of pregnancy? Is he willing to help in the household? Does he possess an understanding and willing self-discipline about sexual activities? Within her environment, the patient's children should be assessed. Do they have the ability to accept the new infant? Has the patient the capacity to accept childhood illness and behavioural difficulties as part of natural parental responsibility. The patient's parents and parents-in-law influence her emotional resources. Did they approve of the marriage, or if they disapproved did they do so in silence? Do they provoke anxiety or resentment between her and her husband, and are they available for emotional support, and physical and financial help when required?

I have tried to draw attention to the importance of careful assessment of the patient. A weakness in one area of emotional resources can be made up by strength in another. Pregnancy is particularly threatening to a patient because it demands adaptation rather than action, and is associated with risks to the health of her baby and herself. The risk of trauma and disability is very real, with an infant mortality of about 2 per cent whilst about 1500 handicapped babies are born in the United Kingdom each week. Following labour there is the assumption of a new role and a new relationship has to be formed involving lactation. Obstetric practice is to identify the patients at high risk and bring sophisticated resources to bear on their care. Antenatal clinics are too large; obstetricians have too little time to discuss with the patient her particular and personal fears and anxieties. If labouring patients are never left alone, it has been found that labours are shorter and less analgesia is required. Where attention is paid to satisfactory bonding between mother and baby, the incidence of rejection, child abuse, and puerperal psychosis has been reduced. It has been clearly shown that patients who have difficult, prolonged, painful labours are less likely to have children in the future.

Obstetric management of mental illness is primarily by prevention, by talking to the patient and allaying her fears and anxieties. When mental illness develops, management depends on understanding the areas of emotional strength which the patient can call upon. Development of severe depression, schizophrenia, hypomania, and mania requires close collaboration with psychiatric colleagues and admission to a psychiatric unit where the staff have experience in dealing with obstetric patients.

4

Neurotic disturbance during pregnancy and the puerperium: preliminary report of a prospective survey of 119 primiparae

R. KUMAR and KAY ROBSON

The incidence of psychotic disorders is increased in the first month or so after labour (Pugh, Jerath, Schmidt, and Reed 1963; Protheroe 1969; see Chapter 6) and while there may be a slight reduction in the occurrence of psychoses during pregnancy, this factor is in itself insufficient to account for the sharp rise after childbirth (Paffenbarger 1964; Kendell, Wainwright, Hailey, and Shannon 1976). Can one discern any similar influences of pregnancy and childbirth on the incidence of less disabling, but very much more common neurotic disturbances, such as states of depression and anxiety?

There is evidence that the incidence of depression is raised during the first few postnatal months (Tod 1964; Pitt 1968; Nilsson and Almgren 1970; Dalton 1971; Kendell *et al.* 1976; Meares, Grimwade, and Wood 1976), but these observations may not be much more accurate or securely based than findings on the incidence of early puerperal psychosis. There are several reasons for this general lack of certainty which are worth detailing here. The collection of 'cases' of puerperal psychosis is typically carried out retrospectively through searches of records of hospital admissions or of case registers, and statistics may vary greatly as a result of disagreements about diagnosis and differences in admission and management policies. It is, however, possible to define operational criteria about what constitutes a case, e.g. admission to mental hospital within a given time after delivery.

Neurotic disturbance during pregnancy and the puerperium:

The adoption of such methods for detecting neurosis would, of course, give a highly distorted picture since most of the relevant subjects would not be admitted to hospital and very few are referred to psychiatric out-patient departments (Shepherd, Cooper, Brown, and Kalton 1966). Determining valid and reliable criteria for defining a 'case' of neurosis is a matter of continuing concern to psychiatrists; direct comparisons between studies of prevalence of neurosis are not easy because of variations in methods of population sampling, data gathering, and evaluation. It does not, therefore, come as a surprise to find that estimates of the incidence of postnatal depression have ranged between 2·9 per cent (20 out of 700 consecutive pregnancies studied by Tod 1964) through 7·5 per cent (14 out of 189 mothers investigated by Dalton 1971) to 10·8 per cent (33 out of 305 mothers studied by Pitt 1968). In a report from Sweden (Nilsson and Almgren 1970), 19 per cent of mothers were thought to have 'clear mental disturbance' post-partum, and although the number of 'new' cases was not specified, about two-thirds of the entire sample (*n* = 152) said that their symptoms had begun, or had become worse, during the first two months post-partum. Meares *et al.* (1976) found that up to 16 per cent of their sample were clinically depressed in the puerperium, but their data were compromised by an extremely high drop-out rate of subjects after delivery.

In their survey of general practice, Shepherd *et al.* (1966) reported that 53 of 341 women who consulted their doctors in connection with pregnancy or the puerperium were noted to be suffering from a psychiatric condition (an annual period prevalence of 15·5 per cent, a rate which did not differ significantly from that for other females aged 45 years or less). About 13 per cent of all the women 'at risk' during the year of this study were regarded as having a 'formal psychiatric illness' and 11·7 per cent fell into the diagnostic category, 'neurosis'. It seems appropriate, therefore, to reopen the question of whether neurotic disturbances really are more common in the puerperium and also formally to assess mental health during pregnancy. This is not merely an academic exercise since the provision of relevant measures

41

of treatment and prevention could have significant implications for mothers at a critical stage of their lives, for the fathers, and, most importantly, for the babies. The ideal investigation would be performed in a large and representative sample of women who had been studied for a time *before* they became pregnant and who would then all be followed through their pregnancies and after childbirth. Comparison with a control group of non-childbearing women would also seem to be indicated, but defining the selection criteria for such a group is likely to be as hard to accomplish as collecting a sample of women who are all about to become pregnant.

The subjects in this serial prospective study were routine attenders at antenatal clinics in a London teaching hospital where, for many years, staff have placed special emphasis on the psychological aspects of motherhood. The women were interviewed at regular intervals both before and after childbirth and vigorous efforts were made to minimize the number of 'drop-outs'. Early in pregnancy, detailed retrospective assessments were also made of each woman's previous mental health, particularly during the three months before she conceived, so that the subject could be used as her own control. The main sample in this study was restricted to primiparae because it was felt that they might more clearly show any impact of pregnancy and childbirth on mental health.

Subjects. 147 women were invited to take part in the survey, the broad aims of which were explained at the outset. The following selection criteria were applied: the subjects should be primiparae whose pregnancies should not have advanced beyond 12–14 weeks; they should be married or have stable relationships with common-law partners (this was to facilitate investigation of changes in marital relationships); they should have spent five of the past ten years in Britain (to ensure an adequate command of English); and, finally, they should live within a reasonable distance of central London.

Eight women declined to participate because of their own or their husband's objections, nine missed or postponed their first interview and could not be contacted again before the 14th week of pregnancy, eight women miscarried, two moved away from London early in pregnancy, and one subject asked to drop out after her initial inclusion in the survey. The sample therefore consisted of 119 primiparae at the start. Four more women moved away from London by the time their babies were three months old and one further subject said she wanted to stop taking part in the study, leaving 114 mothers in the sample at this stage.

Timing of interviews. At about the 12th week of pregnancy, all subjects were first interviewed by a psychologist (K.R.) when they also completed sets of questionnaires. One to two weeks later they were all seen by a psychiatrist (R.K.). They were then all re-interviewed by the psychologist at the 24th and 36th weeks and selected subjects were also seen by the psychiatrist at these times; these were women who had previously been rated as psychiatric 'cases' at the first interview, or were those who subsequently met predetermined screening criteria. All subjects ($n = 114$) were also re-interviewed by the psychiatrist when their babies were about three months old.

Method of clinical assessment. A semi-structured clinical interview schedule (Goldberg, Cooper, Eastwood, Kedward, and Shepherd 1970) was used; this schedule has been found to be particularly suitable for evaluating the nature and severity of recent neurotic disturbance and is being used increasingly in surveys of mental health in the community and in general practice. Ratings of reported symptoms and of manifest abnormalities are made in arriving at a diagnosis and at an assessment of severity which is on a five-point scale—normal (0), mild (1), moderate (2), marked (3), severe (4). A rating of moderate (2) and above constitutes a 'case', i.e. the recent symptoms are judged to have been of pathological severity and to have caused significant distress, at least intermittently. A rating of 'marked' severity roughly

43

corresponds to continuous or severe distress and more obvious manifest abnormalities at interview.

In addition to the clinical interviews, a variety of other questionnaires was administered by the psychologist (K.R.). Of particular relevance here was a detailed structured interview given at 12–14 weeks which gathered personal, historical, and social information, and a personality inventory (Eysenck and Eysenck 1975). At regular intervals, the interviewer also completed check-lists for recent life-events.

The explicit policy of the research workers was not to undertake any treatment in the formal sense, but general advice or reassurance was given if sought. Any medical problems were dealt with by referring subjects back to their family doctors or to an appropriate hospital clinic. The research interviews almost certainly had some therapeutic action and the aim was to optimize conditions for the subjects in the survey. Brief mention will be made in this report of two subsidiary groups of subjects ($n = 38$ primiparae and $n = 40$ multiparae) who participated only in the postnatal part of the survey. By comparing them with the main sample ($n = 119$), we hoped to check whether taking part in the antenatal part of the study might have had some beneficial or preventive action with respect to postnatal depression.

Some characteristics of the main sample. The average age of the group ($n = 119$) was 28 years (range 19–40 years). Eighty-three per cent had been born in the U.K. and about three-quarters belonged to social classes 1, 2, and 3N (i.e. roughly corresponding to upper and middle class groups as judged by husband's occupation; H.M.S.O. 1970). The majority (87 per cent) were in full- or part-time work when first seen. As might be expected, severe financial and housing difficulties were rare. There were no major personal or socio-economic differences between the main ($n = 119$) and the two subsidiary samples ($n = 38$ and $n = 40$). Eighty per cent of the women of the main group ($n = 119$) said they had been trying to become pregnant, 16 per cent reported that, while they had not taken any specific precautions, they had not minded either way about conceiving, and only 4 per cent of the subjects said that their pregnancies had been unplanned. No subject had sought a termination, but 12 per cent (n = 14) had occasionally thought about it. Twenty-nine per cent of this sample (n = 34) had been pregnant at least once before and 21 (18 per cent) had obtained an abortion previously. Five of these women had had both an abortion and a miscarriage and there were 13 subjects who had had one or more miscarriages only. About half the abortions had been done before the Abortion Act 1967 was implemented and seven of the 21 had been illegal.

Previous psychiatric history. Fourteen per cent of the main sample had attended a psychiatrist at least once in the past and a further 13 per cent had received psychotropic drugs from their family doctors for nervous or emotional problems. In the year before they became pregnant, 7 per cent (n = 8) had obtained some sort of psychiatric help (hospital or G.P.), but only three subjects had actually attended a psychiatrist. A retrospective assessment of their mental health in the three months before they became pregnant underlines the generally healthy status of the women in this sample. There had probably been eight 'cases' of neurosis during the three months before pregnancy, seven of whom had recurrent or chronic disturbances (two phobic, one obsessional, and four subjects with depression and/or anxiety); in all seven, the illness had persisted into the first trimester of pregnancy. The eighth subject was probably the only clear 'new' case in the three months before pregnancy; she described a depressive episode which had resolved by about the time she became pregnant.

Neurotic disturbance during early pregnancy. Nineteen cases of neurosis (16 per cent of the sample) were identified at the first clinical interview, including the seven women with chronic disturbances present before pregnancy (see Table 4.1). There were therefore 12 new cases in the first trimester, all with a primary diagnosis of depressive neurosis; this is in sharp contrast with the single new case of depression in the three months before pregnancy (p < 0.01). No instances of

45

Table 4.1 *Prevalence of neurotic disturbance in a group of primiparae before, during, and after pregnancy*

Clinical ratings (severity)	Before pregnancy Retrospective −12 weeks	During pregnancy 12th–14th weeks	24th–36th weeks	Postnatally 12th week
Normal/mild	111	100	107	95
Number of 'cases' moderate/marked	8 (6·7 per cent)	19 (16·0 per cent)	12 (10·1 per cent)	19 (16·7 per cent)
Total number of subjects	119	119	119	114

psychosis were found. In all, there were 15 subjects in the first trimester with a primary diagnosis of depressive neurosis (11 moderate and 4 marked severity) and several of them reported associated symptoms of anxiety; there was one subject with a clinical anxiety state (marked severity). The two cases of phobic disturbance (moderate severity) and one with the obssessive–compulsive disorder (marked severity) continued unchanged throughout pregnancy.

Chi-square tests, t tests, and log-linear models for multiway tables (Bishop, Feinberg, and Holland 1975) were used in order to test associations with the presence of depression and anxiety ($n = 16$ cases) in the first trimester. There was a weak but significant link ($p < 0.05$) with a previous history of consultation or of treatment (hospital or G.P.) for psychological problems. Subjects who were depressed and anxious scored significantly higher than the rest ($p < 0.001$) on the neuroticism dimension of the Eysenck personality inventory (Eysenck and Eysenck 1975); these women were more likely to have occasionally considered terminating the present pregnancy ($p < 0.001$), but such thoughts were transient and occurred as often in subjects who had or had not planned this pregnancy and were independent of a previous history of abortion. Marital tension was also reported more frequently when subjects were depressed ($p < 0.01$). One other important association was between a previous abortion (legal or illegal) and depression and anxiety in early pregnancy. Out of the 21 women who had obtained an abortion at some time in the past, eight were now clinically depressed and/or anxious; of the remaining 98 subjects who had not had previous terminations, only eight were now depressed ($p < 0.001$). Having had a miscarriage did not predispose subjects ($n = 13$) to antenatal depression.

Neurotic disturbance during the second and third trimesters. Thirteen of the 16 women who had been rated initially as being clinically depressed and/or anxious showed clear remission by the second and third trimesters. There were six new cases, all presenting with neurotic depressions (five moderate and one of marked severity) and thus, in total

47

(i.e. including the phobic and obsessional subjects), the prevalence rate for neurotic disturbance between the 24th and 36th weeks was 10·1 per cent (Table 4.1).

All six cases of depression coming to light during the middle and later stages of pregnancy were clearly related to major life-events, such as bereavement or major illness in the close family. We are not able to determine at this stage whether this observation reflects any greater than usual vulnerability to the impact of life-events.

Neurotic disturbance three months after childbirth. The size of the sample was now $n = 114$ and, at the postnatal interview, 19 cases of neurotic disorder were identified; they included four of the women who had been depressed during pregnancy and whose symptoms had either persisted or recurred. There was one obsessional and one phobic subject, the other phobic case having improved spontaneously. There were therefore 13 new cases of depression postnatally.

As before, tests were carried out of possible associations with the presence of postnatal depression in all such cases $(n = 17)$. A relationship with a previous history of psychiatric problems did not now reach statistical significance $(p < 0·1)$ and there was a similar lack of association between high scores obtained antenatally on the neuroticism dimension of the Eysenck personality inventory and postnatal depression $(p < 0·1)$, supporting the view that scores on such tests may in part reflect the present mental state, and diminishing their predictive value (Pitt 1968). Marital tension during pregnancy was related to post-natal depression $(p < 0·01)$ as were original doubts about going through with the pregnancy $(p < 0·01)$. There was a suggestion that subjects who had had difficulties in their relationships with their own parents were now more likely to be depressed $(p < 0·05)$. Finally, two other possibly related factors appeared to contribute significantly $(p < 0·01)$ to the subjects' vulnerability to depression: women who were aged 30 or more years and those who had been trying to conceive for two or more years were more likely to be depressed by the third month after the birth of their first child.

These observations are of a preliminary nature as they have been derived from an ongoing study of women having their first babies. Some of our original aims have largely been met, i.e. we have been able to do a serial prospective study of mental health in women (primiparae) incorporating two major life-events—pregnancy and childbirth. Bias from subjects discontinuing the survey has been kept to a minimum and we have tried to evaluate the therapeutic impact of participation in such a study.

The cumulative prevalence of neurotic disorder in this sample during a period of about six months (twelfth to thirty-sixth weeks of pregnancy) was 21 per cent (25 cases), with a point prevalence in the first trimester of 16 per cent (19 cases; Table 4.1). Differences in methods preclude very direct comparisons, but reference to surveys of women drawn from urban populations (Brown, Bhrolcháin, and Harris 1975) or from attenders in general practice (Shepherd *et al.* 1966; Goldberg, Kay, and Thompson 1976) may suggest that a woman is no more prone to become depressed or anxious if she happens to be pregnant. Simple extrapolations from our particular sample to pregnant women in general could, however, result in appreciable underestimates of the extent of neurotic disorder in pregnancy; this is because our sample turned out to be heavily biased towards the 'healthy' end of the psychosocial spectrum. The subjects were primiparae, all but two of whom were married (selection criteria); the great majority had wanted to become pregnant, most were in stable jobs, and the higher social classes were over-represented. Less than a third had ever had some sort of treatment (hospital or G.P.) for psychological difficulties and only 7 per cent had received such treatment in the past year. The retrospective assessment of the three months before they became pregnant has underlined the generally healthy status of the women in this sample and it also illustrates the impact of pregnancy on mental health as shown by the sharp increase in the incidence of depression in the first trimester.

A previous history of termination of pregnancy is one of several factors which may contribute to an increased vulnerability to depression during early pregnancy; we have described elsewhere (Kumar and Robson 1978) how there appears to be a reactivation of mourning in a proportion of such subjects. It seems, in general, that little attention is paid to the emotional needs of expectant mothers and the problem of antenatal depression (cf. Nilsson and Almgren 1970) merits further investigation.

The lack of a link between antenatal and postnatal depression suggests that there may be rather different patterns of vulnerability at these times, but it may also reflect the therapeutic value of participation in such a survey, i.e. there may have been some degree of resolution of emotional difficulties during pregnancy which might otherwise have persisted into the postnatal period. A comparison of the prevalence of postnatal depression in the main sample ($n = 114$) with the combined subsidiary samples ($n = 79$) provides some support for the hypothesis that taking part in the survey may have reduced the occurrence of postnatal depression. Six of the cases in the subsidiary samples were identified retrospectively and any comparison must therefore be tentative; nevertheless, there were at least 22 depressed women out of 79 in the subsidiary samples as opposed to 17 out of 114 in the main group ($p < 0.05$).

These observations emphasize the need to improve predictors not only of postnatal, but also of antenatal depression and to develop appropriate means of treatment and prevention. It is surprising how few childbearing women either seek or are detected as being in need of help for their emotional problems at a time when they are in repeated contact with the health services.

Professor Herbert Brant and Dr. Elizabeth Tylden have given us invaluable help and advice and we also thank the staff of the Obstetric Hospital, University College Hospital, for their co-operation. Mrs. Frances Campbell and Mrs. Gwyn Macdonald have helped considerably with the interviewing and Mr. Alan Smith with the statistical analyses. Our thanks are due to Professor Sir Denis Hill for his guidance and encouragement, to Professor Michael Shepherd for permission to use and adapt certain questionnaires, and, finally, to the subjects for enduring a great many hours of interviews.

preliminary report of a prospective survey of 119 primiparae

References

Bishop, Y. M. M., Feinberg, S. E., and Holland, P. W. (1975). *Discrete multivariate analysis.* M.I.T. Press, Cambridge, Massachusetts.

Brown, G. W., Bhrolcháin, M. N., and Harris, T. (1975). *Sociology,* 9 225.

Dalton, K. (1971). *Br. J. Psychiat.* 118, 689.

Eysenck, H. J. and Eysenck, S. B. G. (1975). *Manual of the Eysenck personality questionnaire.* Hodder & Stoughton, London.

Goldberg, D. P., Cooper, B., Eastwood, M. R., Kedward, H. B., and Shepherd, M. (1970). *Br. J. prev. soc. Med.* 24, 18.

Goldberg, D., Kay, C., and Thompson, L. (1976). *Psychol. Med.* 6, 565.

Her Majesty's Stationery Office (1970). *Classification of occupations.* London.

Kendell, R. E., Wainwright, S., Hailey, A., and Shannon, B. (1976). *Psychol. Med.* 6, 297.

Kumar, R. and Robson, K. (1978). *Psychol. Med.* in press.

Meares, R., Grimwade, J., and Wood, C. (1976). *J. psychosom. Res.* 20, 605.

Nilsson, A. and Almgren, P. (1970). *Acta psychiat. Scand. Suppl.* 220.

Paffenbarger, R. S. (1964). *Br. J. prev. soc. Med.* 18, 189.

Pitt, B. (1968). *Br. J. Psychiat.* 114, 1325.

Protheroe, C. (1969). *Br. J. Psychiat.* 115, 9.

Pugh, T. F., Jerath, B. K., Schmidt, W. M., and Reed, R. B. (1963). *New Engl. J. Med.* 22, 1224.

Shepherd, M., Cooper, B., Brown, A. C., and Kalton, G. (1966). *Psychiatric illness in general practice.* Oxford University Press, London.

Tod, E. D. M. (1964). *Lancet* ii, 1264.

5

Post-abortion psychosis

C. BREWER

Post-abortion psychosis is a rather emotive subject because abortion itself is still rather emotive. This means that, as with any complication of abortion, those who are opposed to termination of pregnancy have an interest in playing it up while those who wish to see abortion made more easily available have an interest in playing it down. The exact incidence has been difficult to establish because it is only within the last 15 years or so that abortion has been openly performed with any frequency in this country and it is only within the last 10 years that reliable statistics of both NHS and privately performed abortion have been available. Abortion has been more freely available in other countries for a longer period but the results of psychiatric studies in one country or culture, especially where different legal controls may apply, are not necessarily applicable to other countries.

Some early reports indicated a relatively high incidence of psychiatric disturbance following abortion but they were usually anecdotal and involved small numbers. Furthermore they often concerned patients with a previous history of serious psychiatric disturbance and the definitions of psychiatric disorder were often extremely vague, especially in those reports from the U.S.A. where it is now recognized that the diagnosis 'schizophrenia' has been used very loosely and sometimes seems to be almost synonymous with un-American activities.

British psychiatrists, on the whole, were not impressed with the alleged psychiatric dangers of abortion, a notable exception being Sim (1963) who claimed that post-abortion psychosis was 'more malignant' than puerperal psychosis and that there were never any psychiatric grounds for terminating a pregnancy. These comments were published before the first controlled study of post-abortion psychiatric disorder appeared in 1965, when Jansson reported an analysis of psychiatric admissions in one region of Sweden during the period 1952-6. He recorded all admissions to local psychiatric hospitals in which there was a history of a recent legal, illegal, or spontaneous abortion. The total number of legal abortions in the region was known and the number of spontaneous and illegal abortions was estimated. He found that the rate of admission after legal abortion, but not after spontaneous or illegal abortion, was higher than the rate for puerperal psychiatric admissions. However there are two features of this study which make it of dubious relevance to the situation which exists today in countries like Britain with liberal abortion laws. First of all, abortion was still relatively restricted in Sweden at the time of the study and patients with previous psychiatric disorder would have been over-represented. Secondly, the atmosphere of the time may well have led both the psychiatrists and their patients to be somewhat anxious about the possible psychological effects of abortion and this could well have increased the tendency for patients to be admitted. Jansson did set a useful precedent in using admission to a psychiatric ward as the criterion for inclusion in the study. The term, 'psychosis', in the context of the puerperium, generally means psychiatric disorder of sufficient severity to require admission, and clearly the same principle should be used in any comparative study of post-abortion psychosis. This automatically avoids a good deal of argument about the precise meaning of 'psychosis' especially when comparisons are being made with puerperal psychosis in which the clinical picture is often very variable and atypical.

The liberalization of abortion laws in several countries, the existence of reliable abortion statistics, and the increasing similarity of abortion patients to women who carry their pregnancies to term have made a truly comparative study between post-abortion psychosis and post-partum psychosis both possible and necessary. In the United States Tietze and Lewit (1972) followed up to 73 000 abortions and found that the incidence of short-term serious psychiatric sequelae was between 0·2 and 0·4 per 1000 abortions. They too used admission as their main criterion for inclusion but their follow-up period was much less than the traditional three months of the puerperium and there was little information about the mental state and diagnosis of those who were admitted. Nevertheless this study provided strong support for the belief that psychiatric admission was less likely after abortion than after childbirth.

It would be virtually impossible to carry out in Britain a follow-up study involving as many patients as were reported on by Tietze and Lewit (1972) but during 1975 and 1976 I carried out a study (Brewer 1977) very similar to that of Jansson. Twenty consultant psychiatrists in the West Midlands area, as well as the consultant in charge of the regional adolescent unit, agreed to record any admission within three months of a legal abortion. Psychiatric hospitals have defined catchment areas with a known population and the number of legal abortions performed on women normally resident in the West Midlands area is available from official sources. It was thus easy to compute how many abortions would have been performed on the residents of the combined catchment area during the time of the study and the incidence of post-abortion psychosis could therefore be calculated. Since the number of births in the study area was also known, the same technique could be applied to puerperal admissions, and these were also recorded, using similar criteria, for the first three months of the study. Apart from being of interest in itself, this also enabled me to check on the accuracy of the method since if the figure for puerperal admissions had been very different from the usual figures, this would have cast considerable doubt on the validity of the method and hence on the figures for post-abortion admissions. In fact the incidence of puerperal admissions turned out to be 1·7 per 1000 deliveries which is well within the currently accepted range (Jansson 1963).

Although hospital admission was the main criterion for selection, some attempt was made to classify the patients. Post-abortion psychosis was defined as 'a serious disorder requiring admission, and manifesting delusions and/or hallucinations or gross over-activity' occurring within 3 months of legal abortion. Patients were to be further subdivided into two categories depending on whether or not they had a previous history of psychiatric disorder requiring admission to hospital. The instructions made it clear that these categories were intended to embrace 'such diagnoses as mania, schizophrenia, delirium, and the more serious cases of depression'. Consultants were also asked to record any patients who did not satisfy the rather narrow criteria of the two categories above but who had been legally aborted during the previous three months.

From the 3550 legal abortions calculated to have been done on residents of the study area, only a single case of post-abortion psychosis was reported which represents an incidence of 0·3 per 1000 abortions. This is less than one-fifth of the puerperal rate and is encouragingly similar to the American findings. The single case was a woman who had been aborted at an NHS hospital on psychiatric grounds because of two previous puerperal psychoses. These were of essentially depressive type and she had received ECT on both occasions with subsequent recovery. She was aborted by vacuum aspiration at seven weeks and simultaneously sterilized. Ten days after the abortion she was admitted in a depressed state very similar to that during her puerperal admissions and was discharged in a satisfactory condition six weeks later following a further course of ECT. She was followed up for a couple of years after her post-abortion admission and appears to have maintained her recovery. There were no patients in the post-abortion or puerperal group who were thought to qualify for the less serious category.

In addition, I wrote to all 81 consultant adult psychiatrists in the West Midlands region to ask whether they could remember having seen any cases of post-abortion psychosis within the previous two years. Almost half of them replied and only one was able to report such a case which he had seen some 18 months before the start of the study. She was a woman of rather low intelligence who developed an acute and short-lived delusional state within a few days of a legal abortion. She made satisfactory recovery but a year later she became pregnant again and decided to go to term. She was re-admitted at 24 weeks gestation in a moderately depressed state from which she recovered within a month.

The most important potential source of error in this study (as with Jansson's study) is the possibility of a history of recent abortion being overlooked. Certainly it might be easier to miss a recent abortion than a recent delivery but any abortion performed by NHS surgeons would be reported to the referring family doctor and in the region in which the study was carried out most non-NHS abortions were either referred by or notified to family doctors. However the most convincing reason why a history of abortion is in fact unlikely to have been missed is that just as childbirth almost always features in a conversation of women with puerperal illnesses, so it is to be expected that in psychiatric illness related to abortion the fact of the abortion itself would occupy the thought and conversation of the patient, as happened in the two cases reported here.

These results together with the study by Tietze and Lewit (1972) provide very strong evidence that the incidence of serious psychiatric disturbance following abortion is much lower than that following childbirth. There is further circumstantial evidence which also supports this conclusion. First of all we may assume from the official figures that, during the study period, about 350 women in England and Wales were aborted because of a past history of serious psychiatric disorder; yet in this study which covered some 3 per cent of the abortions performed in England and Wales during one year, only one of these 'vulnerable' women came to light when about ten would have been at risk in the study population. Second, although any paper on abortion tends to produce a fair amount of correspondence, nobody wrote to the *British Medical Journal* questioning my interpretation of the results or offering evidence which tended towards a different conclusion. Third, I have carried out a study (Brewer 1978) of women who were aborted by prostaglandins very late in pregnancy after feeling foetal movements. This must surely be as emotionally stressful as it is possible for an abortion to be. At this stage of pregnancy women go through a process of labour very much like those who go to term and they could hardly conceal from themselves that they were acquiescing in the destruction of something very like a small baby. It is interesting that one woman subsequently denied having felt movements even though she was sure enough at the time. The numbers in this study were small and only 25 out of the 40 subjects were followed for three months or more but no trace of serious emotional disturbance occurred and none required any specialist advice.

If, as it seems, the incidence of post-abortion psychosis is much lower than that of post-partum psychosis, I believe that there are certain implications for the aetiology and the treatment of puerperal psychiatric disorders. There seem to be two possible explanations for the difference. On the one hand it could be said that abortion is of trivial emotional importance and that the excess of puerperal psychosis indicates the greater emotional turmoil caused by childbirth and child-rearing, whether welcome or not. This might be supported by some studies which show a greater incidence of puerperal psychosis in the unmarried and by reports of psychosis occurring after the adoption of children.

On the other hand, many people may feel that the termination of an unwanted pregnancy is a more melancholy occasion than the arrival of a wanted child. In most cultures childbirth is a cause for overt rejoicing while abortion—even in this allegedly permissive age—is usually not, and I have yet to be invited to an abortion party. The excess of puerperal psychosis may therefore indicate that hormonal, biochemical, and other 'physiological' changes after childbirth are the major precipitating factors in puerperal psychosis, rather than psychological stress. There have been many studies of biochemical changes in the puerperium and the relationship between post-partum mood and biogenic amines has been discussed in Chapter 2. It seems a reasonable presumption that these changes are much greater after childbirth than after abortion and that this is the main reason why puerperal psychosis is commoner than post-abortion psychosis. If this is the case, and if we can discover which particular bio-chemical changes are the triggers of mental disturbance, it might be possible to treat puerperal psychosis more effec-tively or even to talk in terms of prophylaxis. The obvious differences and similarities between abortion and childbirth represent an interesting and potentially exciting 'natural experiment' for testing a number of hypotheses in this area.

There is actually very little information about the comparative magnitude of post-abortion and post-partum biochemical changes but Dr. Coppen and I are currently studying this question and we hope to be able to report on our findings shortly.

Although I have concentrated on post-abortion *psychosis*, we must not forget that it is possible to be quite seriously dis-turbed and distressed without being admitted to a psychia-tric hospital. It is clear from studies of post-partum mental disorder that many affected women do not seek or do not receive psychiatric help. There is no reason to suppose that abortion is any different in this respect, but at the same time it is almost axiomatic in most conditions that the incidence of less serious complications parallels the incidence of more serious ones. Furthermore the proposition that minor psy-chiatric disturbance is less common after abortion than after childbirth has been confirmed in a number of studies. Whether this reflects primarily psychological or primarily biochemical factors, or both in more or less equal parts, is not known but we hope that the study now in progress and others which it is hoped to carry out may throw some light on this matter as well.

References

Brewer, C. (1977). *Br. med. J.* i, 476.
— (1978). *J. biosoc. Sci.* 10, 203.
Jansson, B. (1963). *Acta. psychiat. Scand.* 39, Suppl. 172.
— (1965). *Acta psychiat. Scand.* 41, 87.
Sim, M. (1963). *Br. med. J.* ii, 145.
Tietze, C. and Lewit, S. (1972). *Studies in Family Planning* 3, 97.

6

A clinical study of
post-partum psychosis

I. F. BROCKINGTON, E. M. SCHOFIELD,
P. DONNELLY, and C. HYDE

The concept of puerperal psychosis, which was one of the
few clearly recognized psychiatric entities during the nine-
teenth century, has in this century almost disappeared from
orthodox thinking. It seems to have been a casualty of the
Kraepelinian diagnostic system. When, at the turn of the century, psychiatrists started to apply the new nosology of
Kraepelin to 'puerperal mania' they found that some patients
belonged to the manic depressive universe and some to dementia praecox, while others had features of toxic confusional or neurotic states, and it was concluded that 'every
reaction type may occur during the puerperium. A puerperal psychosis as a clinical entity does not exist' (Jacobs
1943).

This conclusion, which has had a depressing effect on
research in this area, was based on analyses of hospital
diagnoses made, for the most part, in the U.S.A. Ostwald
and Regan (1957) and Thomas and Gordon (1959) collected
a number of studies, summarized in Table 6.1. Before the end
of the Second World War, a diagnosis of toxic confusional state
was common and seven out of ten studies reported a pre-
ponderance of affective psychoses over schizophrenia. After
that time, the American studies showed an excess of schizophrenia and the British an excess of affective psychoses. The
study of Foundeur, Fixsen, Triebel, and White (1957), for
example, which was carried out in New York claimed that
50 per cent of their patients were schizophrenic, a proportion exactly equalled in the control series of non-puerperal
female admissions. This finding has to be interpreted in the

59

Table 6.1. *Hospital diagnosis made in patients with postpartum psychosis*

	Author	Number of patients	Schizophrenia	Affective psychosis	Toxic psychosis	Other diagnosis
1911	Kilpatrick, U.S.A.	72	14	50	32	4
1911	Runge, Germany	–	37	20	25	–
1924	Gregory, U.S.A.	114	16	46	27	11
1926	Strecker	50	26	36	34	4
1927	Ellery, Australia	89	24	30	44	2
1928	Saunders, U.S.A.	75	60	40	–	–
1928	Stone, U.S.A.	85	45	35	19	1
1933	Anderson, U.K.	50	18	70	8	4
1940	Smalldon, U.S.A.	220	29	49	4	18
1942	Boyd, U.S.A.	150	18	31	29	22
1950	Brew, U.S.A.	83	51	41	5	3
1952	Hemphill, U.K.	140	22	58	–	20
1955	Polonio, Portugal	244	28	3	48	21
1957	Foundeur, U.S.A.	100	50	25	–	25
1958	Martin, Ireland	75	58	37	2	1
1958	Madden, U.S.A.	116	65	15	–	20
1968	Melges, U.S.A.	100	51	31	–	18
1969	Protheroe, U.K.	134	28	67	5	–
1971	Shah, India	102	35	28	12	25
1978	Hyde, U.K. (in preparation)	46	13	21	–	16

Proportion of patients: percentage belonging to various categories light of the now well-known fact that American psychiatrists have a broad concept of schizophrenia embracing most of psychotic illness (Cooper, Kendell, Gurland, Sharpe, Copeland, and Simon 1972). The truth is that hospital diagnostic concepts are far too variable and unstable (geographically and historically) to be capable of resolving a difficult nosological problem such as that of postpartum psychosis, and the studies listed in Table 6.1 leave the status of this disease completely open.

Reading the literature and observing these patients, one forms the impression that in spite of the extreme variability of the clinical picture, there are certain distinctive features. The American psychiatrist James Hamilton, author of *Postpartum psychiatric problems* (1962) described his idea of the typical picture in these terms: 'The onset is relatively acute. There may be evidence of organicity (such as delirium or hallucinations), complaints of fatiguability or diminished responsiveness, and a content appropriate to puerperal patients. The whole pattern of behaviour, including mood, but also thinking and activity, can change very rapidly' (personal communication).

The accuracy of Hamilton's diagnostic clues was demonstrated in a blind diagnostic study of patients admitted to the Mother and Baby Unit at Manchester (Hyde, Hamilton, Monkhouse, Baynes, and Brockington, in preparation). Dr. Hamilton was given transcripts of the mental state and behaviour of 135 patients, including 50 postpartum psychotics, after all non-psychopathological clues to the postpartum state had been removed, and was able to recognize 27 of them, at the expense of 26 false guesses ($P < 0.01$). This provides *prima facie* evidence against the view that these psychoses are completely non-specific.

In this retrospective study, we employed a simple method of psychopathological analysis to search for specific features. In each case, without knowing to which group the patient belonged, we noted the presence or absence of 42 syndromes of disturbed thought, affect or behaviour, mainly taken from Wing's list of 'present state examination syndromes' (Wing, Cooper, and Sartorius 1974). This showed that four of them

61

were significantly commoner in the postpartum group three at the 5 per cent level of probability (agitation, lability of mood, and loss of social reserve) and one at the 1 per cent level ('thought to be clouded or confused').

During the last twenty years improved methods of documenting and diagnosing mental disturbances have been introduced, and we have begun to apply these to puerperal illness. A prospective study of all admissions to the Mother and Baby Unit was begun in 1976 and we have made a preliminary analysis of the results in 26 patients with postpartum breakdowns and 29 non-puerperal psychotic women of the same age group. 'Postpartum psychosis' is defined purely in temporal terms. Paffenbarger (1964) has shown a greatly increased incidence of mental hospital admissions during the first month after delivery, and our retrospective analysis showed that the onset was even more closely related to childbirth, almost all episodes beginning within the first two weeks; accordingly it was defined as an illness leading to admission which began during the first two weeks after parturition. The comparison group were defined by (1) female sex, (2) age 15–37, and (3) the definition of 'psychosis' offered by the *American diagnostic and statistical manual for mental disorders* (1968), which unpublished studies (Brockington and Leff, in preparation) have shown to have a very high agreement with other definitions of psychosis. The methods of study consisted of a mental state inventory conducted with the patient and next-of-kin, a nurse rating schedule, a self-rating questionnaire, and a standardized videotape interview. The schedules included about 200 dichotomous items and 38 visual analogue scales. The analysis proceeded by item-by-item and scale-by-scale comparisons of psychopathology between the puerperal group and controls, and standardized diagnoses derived from the mental state examination via a computer program incorporating some well-recognized operational definitions.

The results have shown a large number of differences between the puerperal group and controls. Of the mental state items, 97 were rated sufficiently often to allow statistical differences to emerge and 6 showed significant differences—

loss of weight, anger, verbal abuse, reduced sociability and poor contact at interview (all commoner in controls), and elation (commoner in puerperal group). The mental state scales showed eight differences—sadness, suicidal ideas, anger, persecution, social withdrawal, poverty of contact and lack of concern (all more severe in the controls), and elation (more severe in the puerperal patients). The fact that 6 of the 97 items showed differences at the 5 per cent level is not impressive, but that 8/38 scales should register differences (3 at the 1 per cent level) supports the view that this psychosis has some specificity. These ratings are, however, open to the objection that they were made by one individual whose observations will have been prejudiced by his views on the nature of puerperal psychosis.

Fortunately, we have two other sources of ratings which are comparatively free from this bias. One of us (P.D.), a medical student serving an elective attachment, reviewed the videotape interviews and rated them with the same 38 visual analogue scales. Eleven scales were eliminated because of low test/retest reliability and 6 of the remaining 27 showed significant differences between the two groups. Passivity experiences, suicidal activity, tension, somatic concern $(P < 0.01)$, and poor self-image $(P < 0.0001)$ were all more severe in the controls; and grandiosity in the puerperal group (elation being more severe in this group too, but unreliably rated). We have also analysed the patients' self-ratings, though in a very small number of puerperal patients (16 against 24 controls), and these have shown four significant differences— suicidal thoughts, self-reference, persecution and social withdrawal all being more severe in the control series.

There must be a good deal of error in these methods which deal mainly with symptoms and not observed behaviour, but certain themes recur. These have been summarized in Table 6.2, which shows that five items are consistently commoner or more severe in the comparison group and one (elation) in the postpartum. Taken with the results of the blind diagnostic study, these are quite strong evidence against the prevailing view that postpartum psychosis is non-specific.

Table 6.2. *Psychopathological difference between postpartum psychoses and controls*

Psychopathology	Worse in	Demonstrated by
Anger	controls	MS items and scale
Elation	postpartum psychosis	MS item and scale
Suicidal ideas	controls	MS scale, SRQ, and video-tape rating
Ideas of persecution	controls	MS scale and SRQ
Reduced sociability	controls	MS item, scale, and SRQ
Poor contact at interview	controls	MS item and scale

MS = mental state examination
SRQ = self-rating questionnaire

The aim of this study is to classify the disease correctly. The prominence of elation and grandiosity suggests that some of these patients were suffering from the manic variety of a bipolar affective illness. There is already some epidemiological evidence which would suggest a special relationship with manic depression. Bratfos and Haug (1966) and Reich and Winokur (1970) have shown that manic depressive women have the same high chance of developing a puerperal psychosis as those women who have already suffered a puerperal breakdown after an earlier pregnancy (1 in 5).

The computer diagnoses summarized in Table 6.3 do indeed show that 10-14 out of 26 patients satisfied operational definitions of mania—a high proportion considering the rarity of manic illness which accounts for less than 10 per cent of psychotic admissions; but our control group also contained a large number of manics and the difference was not statistically significant. As for depressive psychosis, the definition we used, Feighner's affective disorder (Feighner, Robins, Guze, Woodruffe, Winokur, and Munoz 1972), showed a significant excess in controls.

It would be convenient if we could simplify the classification of this disease by eliminating schizophrenia from the range of psychoses associated with the puerperium, thus

Table 6.3. *Computer diagnoses in postpartum psychosis and controls*

Diagnosis	Postpartum psychosis	Controls
Feighner affective disorder	9	20†
Feighner mania	10	5
WHO definition of mania (Leff, Fischer, and Bertelsen 1976)	14	10
Kendell schizoaffective psychosis‡	8	12
Carpenter schizophrenia (6 symptoms)	2	9
Carpenter schizophrenia (5 symptoms)	5	14†
Langfeldt's poor prognosis schizophrenia	7	14
Astrachan's New Haven schizophrenia index	5	8
Spitzer's schizophrenia	4	6
Schneider's first rank symptoms	7	6
Number of patients	26	29

†$P < 0.05$
‡Published by Brockington, Kendell, Kellet, Curry and Wainwright (1978)

allowing it to be identified as an affective psychosis. Our historical review of studies based on hospital diagnosis showed that the idea of puerperal schizophrenia was mainly based on American investigations at a time when they had a very inclusive concept of schizophrenia, and this throws doubt on the association. The results shown on Table 6.3 confirm these doubts to some extent. The definitions of Langfeldt and Carpenter show a difference between the two groups, one of them (Carpenter's 'flexible system' at the threshold of five symptoms present) at the 5 per cent level of statistical significance. Of course, these diagnoses of schizophrenia were based on mental state examination, not a full analysis of the patient's history and course of illness, and we know that such diagnoses can only be made with considerable error. A recent study (Brockington, Kendell, and Leff 1978) has shown that this Carpenter definition, for example, misdiagnosed 25 out of 48 patients in the sense that they showed no further evidence of schizophrenia during the six years' follow-up period, and missed 13 out of 36 patients who did have an outcome diagnosis of schizophrenia.

Operational definitions applied to standardized mental state examinations are an improvement on hospital diagnoses but they do not have the last word in the diagnosis of schizophrenia. A complete psychiatric work-up including a follow-up period is required. It is of interest that the retrospective study of Hyde, Hamilton, Monkhouse, Baynes, and Brockington (in preparation) showed that the outcome of these illnesses was significantly better than that of the control group. Thirty-five made a complete recovery and 15 a partial recovery, compared with 17 full recoveries, 28 partial recoveries, and 5 treatment failures in the controls. If this good prognosis is confirmed, it may further reduce the number of patients ultimately diagnosed as schizophrenic.

There remains one further possibility, namely that postpartum psychosis is a new species of psychiatric illness which shares certain features with the other psychoses because there are only a few ways in which disturbed brain function can be translated into behaviour. In support of this, we have seen a few patients who are hard to classify in Kraepelinian terms. The following is an example of a brief excited state which cleared up more quickly than is usual in mania:

Case 1. Seven days after the birth of her second infant the patient became overactive, 'babbling away sixteen to the dozen and writing pages and pages of absolute rubbish about violence in her marriage'. She was convinced that some of the patients had been planted to spy on her. She lost all her normal shyness, was 'swearing her head off', and at times showed great fear, her hands trembling so much that she could not hold a cup. She seemed confused about time and place but realized that she was having a recurrence of the illness she had after her first baby. Her affect changed rapidly from euphoria to fear. Her motility also varied between extremes. One morning she stood for 15 minutes without moving or saying a word, but in the space of a few hours she was intensely active and talkative. By the sixth day, she had completely recovered and forgotten most of what had happened.

There are others who seem to suffer from extreme mental obfuscation without any evidence of depression.

Case 2. A twenty-year-old primipara was admitted because she could not look after her baby. She said, 'I'm mentally confused. I'm walking about in a dream. I've got to get used to a routine, but I seem to be stuck on one thing. I'll be doing something and my mind will wander onto something else. Thoughts don't come to make conversation. I can't comprehend conversation sometimes. I can't think clearly. I am fed up with being a cabbage and having to be led around.' She was tired and weary but there were no insomnia, suicidal ideas, sadness, or other depressive phenomena. She appeared retarded, especially on cognitive testing, but was fully orientated. She remained in this state for 2–3 weeks and gradually recovered without treatment.

Very careful comparisons of these patients with true manic depressives will be necessary before we can be sure where they belong, and meanwhile the nosological status of postpartum psychosis remains an unsolved problem. The question is an important one. The history of puerperal psychosis illustrates the power of nosology to consign a disease to oblivion; it is hoped that its correct classification will lead to progress in the elucidation of its causes, improved treatment, and, if the association with bipolar illness is confirmed, to new insights into the interaction of neuroendocrine changes with the manic depressive diathesis.

Mrs. Schofield was in receipt of a grant from the North West Regional Health Authority. The Authors would like to thank the consultants and nursing staff at Withington Hospital and Mr. Terry O'Dowd (technical manager) for their help and co-operation.

References

Anderson, E. W. (1933). *J. ment. Sci.* 79, 137.
Astrachan, B. M., Harrow, M., Adler, D., Brauer, L., Schwartz, A., Schwartz, C., and Tucker, G. (1972). *Br. J. Psychiat.* 121, 529.
Boyd, D. A., Jr (1942). *Am. J. Obstet. Gynec.* 43, 148.
Brew, M. and Seidenberg, R. (1950). *J. nerv. ment. Dis.* 111, 408.
Bratfos, O. and Haug, J. O. (1966). *Acta psychiat. Scand.* 42, 285.
Brockington, I. F., Kendell, R. E., and Leff, J. P. (1978). *Psychol. Med.* (in press).
——— Kellet, J. M., Curry, S. H., and Wainwright, S. (1978). *Br. J. Psychiat.* (in press).
Carpenter, W. T., Strauss, J. S., and Bartko, J. J. (1973). *Science, N.Y.* 182, 1275.
Cooper, J. E., Kendell, R. E., Gurland, B. J., Sharpe, L., Copeland, J. R. M., and Simon, R. (1972). *Psychiatric diagnosis in New York and London.*
Ellery, R. S. (1927). *Med. J. Aust.* 1, 287.
Feighner, J. P., Robins, E., Guze, S. B., Woodruffe, R. A., Winokur, G., Munoz, R. (1972). *Arch. gen. Psych.* 26, 57.

Foundeur, M., Fixsen, C., Triebel, W. A., and White, M. A. (1957). *Arch. Neurol. Psychiat.* 77, 503.

Gregory, M. S. (1924). *Am. J. Obstet. Gynec.* 8, 420.

Hamilton, J. A. (1962). *Postpartum psychiatric problems.* Mosby, St. Louis.

Hemphill, R. E. (1952). *Br. med. J.* 48, 1232.

Jacobs, B. (1943). *J. ment. Sci.* 89, 242.

Kilpatrick, E. and Triebout, H. M. (1926). *Am. J. Psychiat.* 6, 145.

Langfeldt, G. (1960). *Proc. roy. Soc. Med.* 53, 1047.

Leff, J. P., Fischer, M., and Bertelsen, A. (1976). *Br. J. Psychiat.* 129, 428.

Madden, J. J., Luhan, J. A., Tutex, W., and Bimmerle, J. F. (1958). *Am. J. Psychiat.* 115, 18.

Martin, M. E. (1958). *Br. med. J.* ii, 773.

Melges, F. T. (1968). *Psychosom. Med.* 30, 1.

Ostwald, P. F. and Regan, P. F. (1957). *J. nerv. ment. Dis.* 125, 153.

Paffenbarger, R. S. (1964). *Brit. J. prev. soc. Med.* 18, 189.

Polonio, P. and Figueiredo, M. (1955). *Mschr. Psychiat. Neurol.* 130, 304.

Protheroe, C. (1969). *Br. J. Psychiat.* 115, 9.

Reich, T. and Winokur, G. (1970). *J. nerv. ment. Dis.* 151, 60.

Runge, W. (1911). *Arch. Psychiat.* 2, 645.

Saunders, E. B. (1929). *Am. J. Psychiat.* 8, 669.

Schneider, K. (1959). *Clinical psychopathology*, pp. 133–4. Grune and Stratton, London and New York.

Shah, D. K., Wig, N. N., and Akhter, S. (1971). *Indian J. Psychiat.* 13, 14.

Smalldon, J. R. (1940). *Am. J. Psychiat.* 98, 80.

Strecker, E. and Ebaugh, F. (1926). *Arch. Neurol. Psychiat.* 15, 239.

Stone, C. W. and Karnosh, L. J. (1928). *Ohio State med. J.* 24, 29.

Thomas, C. L. and Gordon, J. E. (1959). *Am. J. med. Sci.* 238, 363.

Wing, J. K., Cooper, J. E., and Sartorius, N. (1974). *The measurement and classification of psychiatric symptoms.* Cambridge University Press, London.

7

Childbirth as an aetiological agent

R. E. KENDELL

At one time puerperal psychosis was believed to be a distinct form of insanity with a symptomatology, psychopathology, and prognosis different from those of other psychoses. But the demonstration a generation ago that the clinical features and the prognosis of puerperal illnesses were both much the same as those of other functional psychoses (Vislie 1956; Foundeur, Fixsen, Triebel, and White 1957) discredited this belief. As a result, interest in the concept of puerperal psychosis waned and contemporary psychiatric glossaries discourage use of the term. None the less, there is good evidence that childbirth is followed by a sharp rise in the incidence of functional psychoses. Pugh, Jerath, Schmidt, and Reed (1963), for example, studied admissions of women of childbearing age to public mental hospitals in Massachusetts and found that, although the admission rate was below expectation throughout pregnancy, it rose to several times the expected rate in the first three months after delivery. As this rise was too large to be accounted for by the postponement of illnesses (or admissions) that would normally have occurred during pregnancy, Pugh's findings strongly suggest that childbirth is a genuine causal factor in the genesis of psychosis. It remains unclear however whether the crucial influences are psychological or somatic. Some authors have found a raised incidence of first pregnancies and stillbirths in women developing puerperal psychoses and interpreted this as evidence of psychogenesis; others, like Paffenbarger (1964), have found a raised incidence of obstetric complications of various kinds and regarded these as evidence of a somatic basis.

The pilot study described here was carried out at the Institute of Psychiatry in 1973–74 with the help of Mrs. Sue Wainwright, Dr. Anthea Hailey, and Mrs. Barbara Shannon. Its design was similar to that of Pugh *et al.* (1963) except that we studied a wider range of illness—out-patients as well as in-patients—in a smaller population. In fact the study was based on data accumulated by the Camberwell Psychiatric Register—a record of all psychiatric contacts from 1965 onwards, either as in-patient, out-patient, or ward referral, by the 174 000 inhabitants of the former London Borough of Camberwell (now part of Southwark).

All women resident in the catchment area of the Camberwell register giving birth to children in 1970 were identified by searching through the live and still-birth registers of the adjacent boroughs of Southwark, Lambeth, and Lewisham, and extracting all those with addresses in Camberwell. These women, and their husbands, were then sought in the files of the case register and note made of any psychiatric contact in the two years before or the two years after the birth of the child. This four-year period was arbitrarily divided into sixteen trimesters, with the starting date of each calculated from the exact date of childbirth (i.e. with the 9th trimester starting the day after childbirth). Separate new and repeat consultation rates were calculated for each of these trimesters, in mothers and fathers separately, for mental illness as a whole and also for various diagnostic categories individually.

Fifteen still births and 2242 live births to women resident in the register catchment area were traced. A search through the register files for these 2257 mothers and 2116 fathers (no father was recorded on 141 birth certificates) produced 99 mothers and 39 fathers with one or more psychiatric contacts within the four-year period in question.

The distribution of psychiatric contacts relative to the time of childbirth was studied in these men and women with the main focus of interest on the timing of 'new episodes', a new episode being defined as any psychiatric contact, either as an in- or out-patient, not preceded by any other contact in the previous three months. In fact the majority were out-patients; only 24 of the mothers and nine of the fathers were admitted to a psychiatric hospital during the study period.

The total numbers of mothers and fathers under psychiatric care each trimester, and the corresponding 'new episode' rates, are set out in Table 7.1, and shown as histograms in Fig. 4. In the fathers the total number in treatment and the new episode rate are both low and do not show any significant variation with time (chi square = 9·02 and 13·58 respectively and $p > 0.5$ for both). In the mothers the situation is very different. Both rates are higher throughout, and both show a prominent peak in the three-month period immediately after childbirth and a more prolonged rise later on. This variation with time is highly significant (chi square = 29·50

Table 7.1. *Total 'in treatment' and 'new episode' rates per trimester in mothers and fathers—all diagnoses combined*

Trimester	Mothers		Fathers	
	In treatment	New episodes	In treatment	New episodes
1	13·3	6·1	8·6	2·5
2	16·7	11·9	13·3	7·3
3	18·7	12·9	10·6	3·5
4	13·7	5·7	8·1	2·3
5	13·4	10·1	7·9	1·1
6	13·1	10·9	8·8	5·5
7	7·4	3·2	7·5	2·1
8	9·3	9·3	8·3	3·1
9	25·8	22·7	10·4	5·2
10	19·1	7·4	8·6	3·2
11	13·1	6·5	9·9	6·6
12	22·4	15·7	12·4	4·5
13	22·8	13·7	10·4	3·5
14	28·1	11·7	13·0	4·7
15	21·4	10·7	8·5	2·4
16	18·2	7·3	3·7	1·2

Note: These figures have been 'corrected' to allow for the effects of migration across the register boundary. Although everyone was resident in Camberwell at the time the birth certificate was issued, some families would have entered the district within the previous two years, or left within the following two, and any contacts before entering or after leaving would not be recorded in the register. The extent of this migration was estimated from 1971 census data.

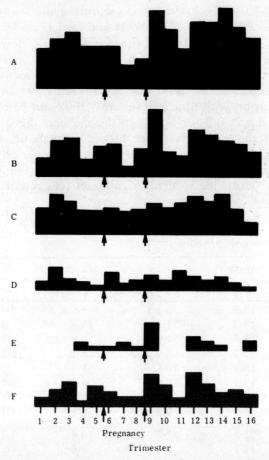

FIG. 4. Corrected 'in treatment' and 'new episode' totals per trimester. Key: (A) Mothers—total in treatment; (B) Mothers—all new episodes; (C) Fathers—total in treatment; (D) Fathers—all new episodes; (E) Mothers—new episodes of functional psychosis; (F) Mothers—new episodes of depressive illness.

and $p < 0.02$ for all contacts; chi square $= 31.68$ and $p < 0.01$ for new episodes).

The contribution made by different diagnostic categories to this overall rise is shown in Table 7.2, and in histogram form in Fig. 4. New episodes of functional psychosis show a dramatic peak in the 9th trimester (chi square $= 49.18$ and

Table 7.2. *'Corrected' new episode rates per trimester in mothers—by diagnosis*

Trimester	Functional psychoses	Depressive illnesses	Anxiety states	Illegitimate births —all diagnoses
1	—	2·4	2·4	1·2
2	—	4·8	2·4	3·6
3	—	8·2	—	3·5
4	2·3	1·1	—	2·3
5	1·1	6·7	2·2	—
6	1·1	4·4	3·3	3·3
7	2·1	3·2	—	—
8	1·0	3·1	—	1·0
9	9·2	11·3	3·1	6·2
10	—	7·4	—	2·1
11	—	3·3	2·2	2·2
12	4·5	12·3	2·2	3·4
13	2·3	8·0	3·4	1·1
14	1·2	4·7	5·9	1·2
15	—	6·0	1·2	3·6
16	3·6	4·8	—	1·2
Uncorrected totals	26	82	25	32

$p < 0.0001$). There were in fact nine new psychotic episodes in the 9th trimester, compared with seven in the whole of the preceding two years. Of these nine illnesses, seven were depressive, one manic, and one schizophrenic, the last being in a woman who had had schizophrenic breakdowns at least twice before. Seven of these nine women came under psychiatric care within three weeks of delivery and, as Table 7.2 shows, there were no new episodes of psychosis in either the 10th or the 11th trimesters, suggesting that psychotic illnesses attributable to childbirth develop within a few weeks of the event. Depressive illnesses as a whole (i.e. psychotic and neurotic illnesses combined) also show a peak in the 9th trimester and a second slightly higher peak in the 12th. Again, the variation with time is significant, though less strikingly so than for the functional psychoses (chi square $= 25.40$ and $p < 0.05$).

It is apparent from Tables 7.1 and 7.2, and also from the histograms in Fig. 4, that, quite apart from the high new episode rates in the 9th trimester, there is a general tendency for all rates to be higher after childbirth than before it. If one takes the average rate in the first five trimesters as the base rate before the onset of pregnancy and then compares this with the average rate in the last five trimesters, the latter is consistently higher, both for new episodes and all contacts, and for all diagnostic categories separately. The difference between the two is only statistically significant for all contacts by mothers ($t = 3.84$, $d.f. = 4$, and $p < 0.02$), but the steadily rising trend of the CuSum plots shown in Fig. 5 is suggestive of a sustained increase in new episode rates also. (CuSum plots are a convenient way of illustrating, and detecting, changes in base rates. Originally developed as an aid to industrial quality control, they are simply a plot of the accumulated sum of the differences between the rate for each successive time period and the average rate (k) over a previous time span. Here k is based on the five trimesters before the start of pregnancy, so the CuSum plot represents the cumulative divergence from the average new episode rate before pregnancy.) The rising slope of these plots between the 10th and the 16th trimesters suggests that, not only is there a considerable increase in the number of mothers *under psychiatric care* after childbirth, but also that there may be a persistent rise in the *incidence* of psychiatric illness, particularly affective illness (i.e. depressions and anxiety states) over and above the initial increase in the first three months after delivery.

The 99 mothers who developed a 'new episode' of psychiatric illness in the four-year study period were compared with the 2158 who did not. There were no significant differences in the sex ratio of their offspring or in the mothers' country of birth (63 per cent of both groups were born in the U.K. and the rest mainly in the West Indies (15 per cent) or Eire (8 per cent)). There was, however, a significant excess of illegitimate births in the study population—22·2 per cent, compared with 11·1 per cent overall (chi square = 10·19 and $p < 0.01$). Finally, the 21 mothers who developed a

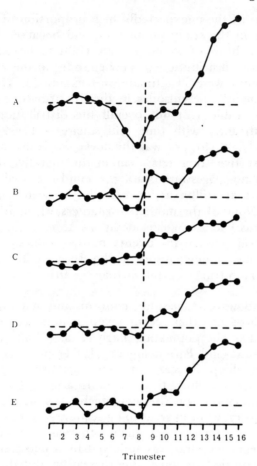

FIG. 5. CuSum plots to illustrate changes in base rates (in mothers). Key: (A) Total in treatment; (B) All new episodes; (C) New episodes of functional psychosis; (D) New episodes of depressive illness; (E) New episodes of affective illness (depressions plus anxiety states).

'new episode' in the 9th trimester (i.e. immediately after childbirth) were compared with the 78 who only developed new episodes at other times in the four-year study period. The only significant difference to emerge was that a higher proportion of the former were born outside the U.K. (12 of 21 compared with 24 of 78; chi square = 3·90 and $p < 0.05$).

75

Because of the unexpectedly high proportion of illegitimate births in the study population, and because one might expect the birth of an illegitimate child to be particularly stressful, the distribution of new episodes in the 22 women whose babies were illegitimate was examined. There were twice as many new episodes in the 9th trimester as in any other (see Table 7.2) but overall the distribution did not vary significantly with time (chi square $= 17 \cdot 64$ and $p <$ $0 \cdot 2$ with $d.f. = 15$), nor was the new episode rate any higher in the last five trimesters than in the first five. Similarly, there was no suggestion, bearing in mind the small numbers available, that stillbirths or twin births were particularly stressful. None of the mothers, or fathers, of the fifteen still-born infants had a new episode at any time in the four-year study period. Two of the twenty mothers who gave birth to twins did have a new episode in the study period, but in the 11th and 16th trimesters rather than the 9th.

The findings of this study confirm, and in some respects extend, those of other recent investigations. These London mothers, like the population Pugh *et al.* (1963) studied in Massachusetts and Paffenbarger's (1964) patients in Ohio, showed a sharp increase in new episodes of functional psychosis in the first three months after delivery. As in Pugh's population, this rise was largely attributable to affective psychoses, was too great to be accounted for by the postponement of illnesses that might otherwise have developed during pregnancy, and was followed by a persistent though less dramatic rise for some time thereafter. But the effect of childbirth is not restricted to psychotic illness. 'Post-partum blues' is familiar to most obstetricians and general practitioners and those who have investigated the phenomenon, like Ryle (1961), Tod (1964), and Pitt (1968), have all found an inordinately high incidence of relatively mild depressions in the puerperium. Here too there was a clear-cut rise in the new episode rate after delivery for all diagnostic categories combined and for all depressions, not just for functional psychoses. In the fathers, however, the event produced no rise in the new episode rate, or even in the consultation rate.

76

Perhaps this is not surprising, but it does suggest that the Couvade syndrome (psychiatric disturbance in men during their wives' pregnancy or confinement) is not a particularly widespread phenomenon.

A high proportion of the 99 women who developed new episodes of psychiatric illness during the four-year study period gave birth to illegitimate children—22 per cent compared with 11 per cent in the parent population. However, the 22 mothers concerned had no more new episodes in the last five trimesters of the study period than in the first five and, although they did show a raised new episode rate in the ninth trimester, this was no greater than in the mothers of legitimate children. It is clear therefore that the relationship between an illegitimate pregnancy and psychiatric illness is not a simple matter of cause and effect. The two are associated, but the psychiatric disorder is as likely to precede as to follow the illegitimate pregnancy, suggesting that both are attributable to some third variable, probably the woman's personality, or her social environment, or the interaction of the two.

There are few clues from the results of this study, or from the literature, to the cause of the raised incidence of psychiatric illness in the puerperium. It is worth noting, however, that several events which one might expect to be particularly stressful psychologically—stillbirths, illegitimate births, and twin births—all failed to produce any increased risk of puerperal illness. Nor was there any evidence of increased morbidity in the fathers, who of course share with their wives at least some of the psychological stresses of childbirth, but none of the somatic ones.

Finally, there is the suggestion of a secondary rise in the new episode rate from the twelfth to the sixteenth trimesters (i.e. from nine to twenty-four months after delivery) to consider. The birth of a child, particularly a first child, may be stressful in many different ways—by forcing the mother to stop work and keeping her at home, by reducing the family income, by necessitating a change of housing, and above all by committing her to a task for which she may have little talent or inclination. It may be, therefore, that this secondary rise is produced by a *mélange* of different factors of this kind quite distinct from the unknown influences responsible for the initial puerperal rise. It would have been very informative to have compared the distribution of new episodes in the two-year period after childbirth in primigravidae and multigravidae, as it is likely that the initial psychological stress and subsequent changes in life style are both considerably greater in the former than the latter, but, although this information is routinely recorded on birth certificates, the Population (Statistics) Acts forbid its disclosure.

I started by describing this investigation as a pilot study and I hope that the implication of this—that there is a larger and better designed study to follow—will be fulfilled. As it stands this study has several shortcomings. Because birth registers rather than hospital records were used as the primary data source it was not possible to distinguish between primigravidae and multigravidae, or to assess the influence of obstetric variables like toxaemia or prematurity. Secondly, the cohort was too small to generate adequate instances of uncommon events like stillbirths and twin births, with the result that no firm conclusions can be drawn about the incidence of psychiatric disorder associated with these. Most important of all—and this is a shortcoming shared by all previous investigations—the study was based only on consultations with psychiatrists. Consequently the possibility remains that the observed rise in the incidence of psychiatric disorder after childbirth is spurious and that all that really changes after delivery is that women who previously tolerated their depressive symptoms, or consulted other doctors, no longer do so afterwards but consult, or are referred to, psychiatrists instead.

Dr. J. L. Cox and I in Edinburgh are trying to remedy these deficiencies. Since last year Edinburgh has had a psychiatric case register in operation, similar to the Camberwell Register but covering all 470 000 inhabitants of the city. This enables us to mount a larger-scale study than was possible in Camberwell. We will also be able to obtain comprehensive information about all births in Edinburgh directly from the returns made by the five obstetric units in the city to the

Home and Health Department and so gain immediate access to a wealth of obstetric data. We are also in the process of obtaining serial ratings of mood, derived partly by questionnaire and partly by clinical interview, from a cohort of several hundred women at various stages during pregnancy and the puerperium, and these should enable us to determine whether the dramatic changes in psychiatric consultation rates observed after delivery are accompanied by corresponding changes in symptomatology.

This study is described in more detail in *Psychol. Med.* 6, 297–302 (1976). The editor is grateful to the Cambridge University Press for permission to reproduce the diagrams and parts of the text from that article.

References

Foundeur, M., Fixsen, C., Triebel, W. A., and White, M. A. (1957). *Arch. Neurol. Psychiat.* 77, 503.

Paffenbarger, R. S. (1964). *Brit. J. prev. soc. Med.* 18, 189.

Pitt, B. (1968). *Br. J. Psychiat.* 114, 1325.

Pugh, T. F., Jerath, B. K., Schmidt, W. M., and Reed, R. B. (1963). *New Engl. J. Med.* 268, 1224.

Ryle, A. (1961). *J. ment. Sci.* 107, 279.

Tod, E. D. M. (1964). *Lancet* ii, 1264.

Vislie, H. (1956). *Acta psychiat. neurol. Scand.* Suppl. 111.

8

Hormones and post-partum depression

MICHAEL GELDER

The idea that puerperal mental illness has a physiological cause is not new. In 1835, Prichard discussed in his textbook the theory that the normal redistribution of the circulation from uterus to breasts, which was assumed to take place in the first days' after delivery, might be disturbed, with a consequent change in blood flow to the brain—and hence mental disorder. With greater knowledge of physiology these ideas are easily dismissed, but they are nevertheless important because they prompt us to ask whether the present hormonal theories are any better founded. For this reason, I shall begin with a summary of the endocrine changes which have been shown to take place between late pregnancy and the early puerperium.

This is a subject of great complexity and many uncertainties. The account which follows is necessarily brief and oversimplified, but it is sufficient to demonstrate some of the problems which beset attempts to relate hormonal changes to mental disturbance. A particular difficulty is that, almost invariably, the published data refers only to pregnancy. Observations are not carried out in the puerperium, presumably because the investigations have been mainly concerned with foeto-placental physiology and with the mechanism of labour.

The most striking changes, and those which have received most attention in relation to mental illness, are in oestrogens and progesterone. Figures 6 and 7 show the changes which we recorded in a group of women whose mental state was also being studied (Nott, Franklin, Armitage, and Gelder 1976). They show the well-known precipitous fall in

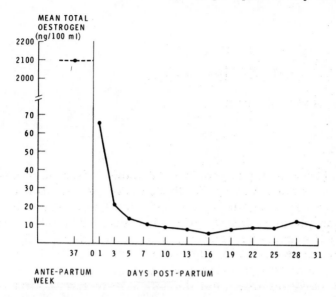

FIG. 6. Changes in mean total oestrogen levels in the plasma between the last month of pregnancy and the end of the first month post-partum. (Redrawn from data of Nott *et al.* 1976).

circulating total oestrogen and in progesterone over the first few days of the puerperium. These striking changes invite speculation that mental disturbances might result from a failure of adjustment; indeed it might be argued that it is the normal adjustment to such sudden alterations in hormone levels which is remarkable, rather than an occasional failure.

These are not, of course, the only changes. There are complicated alterations in adrenal steroids as well (Cope 1972). Total plasma 17-hydroxycorticosteroids increase throughout pregnancy to reach levels just before delivery which are about twice the normal. However, this change is accompanied by a doubling of corticosteroid binding globulin from 35 to 70 mg/l probably as a response to rising oestrogen levels. The net result is an increase in morning levels of free cortisol from 0·67 to 1·4 ng/100 ml. However, Burke and Roulet (1970) have shown that matters are even more complex because control of day/night rhythm in late pregnancy alters in

81

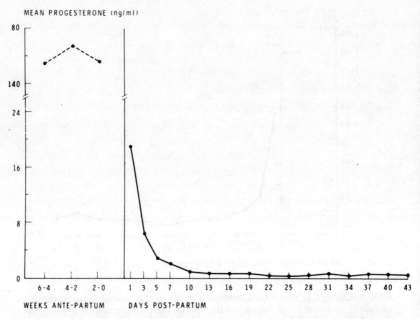

FIG. 7. Changes in plasma progesterone between the last month of pregnancy and the end of the first month post-partum. (Redrawn from data of Nott *et al.* 1976).

such a way that midnight levels are greater in proportion to those at 9.00 a.m. than they are in women who are not pregnant. Although levels of free cortisol return to normal soon after delivery, little is known about the readjustments of hypothalamic control of day/night rhythm, or of changes which take place in the proportions of free and bound cortisol as binding globulin and total 17-hydroxycortico-steroids find new levels; still less is known about individual differences in these adjustments.

Because both thyrotoxicosis and hypothyroidism are sometimes followed by mental disorder, it has also been suggested that thyroid hormones are involved in puerperal mental disorders. However, although the placenta produces a TSH, free levels of T_3 and T_4 show little change in pregnancy —though T_4-binding globulin and total T_4 do rise. The increase in binding globulin is in turn related to high oestrogen

82

levels in the mother. Individual differences in the readjustment of these hormones in the puerperium have not been studied.

There is no space here to discuss changes in prolactin, the gonadotrophins, or other hormones during pregnancy and the puerperium. However, enough has been presented to indicate the complexity of the changes and the naivete of most of the hormonal theories of puerperal mental disturbance which we are about to review.

Before turning to the clinical syndromes of post-partum depression, it is appropriate to consider what sort of evidence would confirm or refute the hypothesis that an abnormality in a particular hormone causes mental disorder. It is helpful to begin by considering the circumstances in which definite endocrine disorder is followed by mental symptoms.

Psychoses may appear in disorders of thyroid or adrenal function, as well as during treatment with adrenal steroids. In these circumstances it has been observed that the form of mental disorder is not specific to the endocrine state. It is also clear that there is no difference in the severity of the endocrine disorder or dosage schedule of steroid treatment, between those who develop psychiatric symptoms and those who do not. And finally, the psychosis often persists after endocrine balance has been restored, and requires treatment with antidepressant or neuroleptic drugs.

It follows that while the demonstration of endocrine differences between women who are depressed and those who are not would be evidence for an endocrine cause, failure to show a difference would not rule it out. Nor would the absence of a therapeutic response to hormones settle the point. The theory, like many others which persist in psychiatry, cannot be disproved; it can only wait to be confirmed.

Other chapters in this book have reviewed the mental disorders which appear in the puerperium. Much of the literature on hormones and mental disturbance is confused because the authors fail to indicate clearly what range of clinical phenomena they are attempting to explain. For our purposes, it is convenient to divide the material into three: severe depressive illnesses (depressive psychoses), transient

minor affective disturbances ('maternity blues'), and an inter-
mediate group of depressive disorders of moderate degree
and variable extent. Since each has been discussed elsewhere, the sections which follow will refer only to features
of these states which are relevant to their possible relationship to hormonal disturbances. In doing so, no attempts
will be made to give complete references to the literature.

Hormones and minor affective disturbance. The striking
way in which 'maternity blues' cluster round the third post-
partum day, and the frequency with which they appear, has
led to much speculation about hormonal causes. The conditions are observed in about half the women who are delivered
(estimates vary according to the criteria of diagnosis. Some
of the clinical features appear to be in keeping with an
'organic' cause. Thus, irritability, mood lability, and poor
sleep are all common and are somewhat similar to symptoms
which are observed after withdrawal of a sedative drug;
and progesterone in very large doses has sedative effects in
animals (Gyermark, Genther, and Fleming 1967). Further,
the supposed occurrence of confusional symptoms has been
put forward as rather strong evidence for an organic cause
(Yalom, Lunde, Moos, and Hamburg 1968). However, while
patients often complain that they feel confused in the everyday sense of that word, when tests of concentration were
given no objective changes were found to support this (Nott
et al. 1976). At first sight, therefore, the clinical phenomena
lend some support to the idea of an endocrine cause. As well
as changes in oestrogens and progesterone (Malleson 1953;
Yalom *et al.* 1968), abnormalities in corticosteroids (Bower
and Altschule 1956) have been suggested.

Unfortunately, many of these ideas about hormones are
based on doubtful assumptions about the natural course of
the condition. They take for granted that depression begins
after childbirth. However, when patients have been studied
as carefully before delivery as afterwards, it has been found
that the group who rate themselves most depressed in the
first few post-partum days were reporting equally high levels
of depression in the last weeks of pregnancy (Nott *et al.*

1976; Davidson 1972). When evidence is sought even earlier in pregnancy, it is found that depression is as common in the first trimester as in the last (Lubin, Gardener, and Roth 1975). All these observations indicate the need for more precise clinical studies to determine which symptoms observed in the puerperium are arising anew, and which have carried over from pregnancy. While there might be a hormonal component to the aetiology of either, little progress is likely until they can be examined separately.

As there was no study which had measured female hormones in 'blues' patients we decided to perform one (Nott *et al.* 1976). In order to increase the chances of identifying hormonal effects if such exist, we investigated patients who gave no history of previous psychiatric disorder and had no major social difficulties. Blood samples were taken for hormonal estimations three times before delivery and 16 times afterwards. Patients were divided into two groups according to their scores on a 'blues' questionnaire (Pitt 1968). Using this criterion, 13 patients had 'blues' and 14 did not. When hormonal measures were compared in these two groups, no significant differences were found either before or after the delivery in progesterone, total oestrogen, oestrogen/progesterone ratio, LH, FSH, and prolactin.

Because many patients who reported blues in the puerperium had also reported similar symptoms before delivery, we examined in more detail three symptoms which we thought particularly characteristic of the 'blues'. These were: emotional lability, poor sleep, and irritability. Measures of oestrogen and progesterone were then correlated with ratings of the questionnaire items which were concerned with these symptoms. No correlations were found which reached an acceptable level of significance. However the negative correlation between progesterone changes and sleep disturbance is the opposite to that predicted by the progesterone–sedation hypothesis. Changes in this hormone also failed to correlate with irritability. Despite these negative findings, the general method of analysing the problem could be used profitably in a future study using better methods to separate mood disturbances starting at the puerperium from those which have

85

carried through from pregnancy, as well as more complete endocrine measurements.

We also examined whether any factors in the patients' history correlated with the appearance of the 'blues' syndrome. We found, as others have done, that there was no relation to obstetric or anaesthetic complications at the time of delivery. We also found, in keeping with the findings of Yalom *et al.* (1968), that 'blues' are more common in primiparous women. 'Blues' patients were also more likely to report premenstrual tension, a point also noted by Yalom *et al.* It is not clear whether this last finding indicates that some women are particularly susceptible to changes in female hormone concentrations whenever they occur, or whether it merely reflects the threshold at which women begin to report minor degrees of discomfort.

Before further elaborate endocrine measurements are carried out—e.g. of free and bound hormones—it is essential to improve the clinical description of patients, separating cases in the way we have described. A somewhat similar point was made by Meares, Grimwade, and Wood (1976) although their attempt to study it was unsatisfactory because it was retrospective. At the same time it may be fruitful to examine further the middle trimester of pregnancy when depression is reported to be relatively uncommon (Lubin *et al.* 1975). While these clinical studies are proceeding, further endocrine studies are required to examine in detail the readjustment in hormone levels immediately after delivery and the extent to which there are individual differences in this. Until we have more precise information of this kind, hormonal theory will continue to be mere speculation.

Depressive psychoses in the puerperium. These rare but striking disorders have also attracted much speculation about hormonal causes. We shall see that the evidence for this is even weaker than that for the 'blues' syndrome. Puerperal psychoses appear only once or twice in every thousand births. They begin, usually, between the third post-partum day and the end of the second week and this timing is one of the points which has suggested a hormonal cause. The condition can take the form of schizophrenia as well as depressive illness, the proportion of these types being about the same as that seen in women of the same age who are not pregnant. Moreover, the little evidence which is available suggests that in regard to personal and family history, women who develop post-partum psychoses resemble other psychotic patients more closely than they resemble normal women (Seager 1960). All this suggests that if hormonal changes have importance, it is only as a factor which provokes a psychosis in a predisposed person.

One set of observations suggests that if there is a hormonal cause it may not be one which is specific to pregnancy. Stengel, Zeitlyn, and Rayner (1958) have pointed out that two features which have been claimed to be specific to puerperal psychoses are also seen quite commonly in post-operative mental disorders. These are confusion in the early days of the illness (Jansson 1964), and a mixture of schizophrenic and affective symptoms appearing at the same time. Stengel *et al.* also remind us that the two-day latent period commonly described in puerperal psychoses is observed rather frequently among post-operative cases. It might be thought unwise to add to the speculation about this subject; however, these observations do suggest that it may be fruitful to look particularly carefully at factors common to the puerperium and the post-operative state. Of these, changes in adrenal steroids suggest themselves. The increase in plasma corticosteroid levels immediately before and during operations, and their subsequent fall are not, of course, the same as the changes with childbirth. However, the readjustments in cortisol production, excretion, and in binding globulins are sufficiently complex to make it plausible that considerable differences could arise between subjects in the resultant levels of free cortisol and that these anomalies might arise in both clinical states. Such speculations are not new; they were put forward in a somewhat different form by Bower and Altschule (1956) and by Hamilton (1962). It is clear that research could usefully be directed to the pattern of individual differences in the readjustments of adrenal function after childbirth.

Hormones and moderate depressive disorders. This is the group of disorders in which hormonal causes are least plausible. It is also the group which has been described least precisely by clinicians. Depression may start at any time after delivery, often after the patient has returned home, and may last from a few weeks to many months. Some cases cannot be separated clearly from an initial intense episode of maternity blues, but many begin later and seem more clearly related to the psychological adjustments of motherhood and the burdens of bringing up the new baby. About one woman in ten appears to suffer depression of this kind and about 4 per cent persist for as long as a year. The variable course of the illness reminds us that in minor states of depression it is important to think not only of the factors which start the disorder, but also of those which prevent its rapid resolution. Sociologists such as Brown, Harris, and Peto (1973) have emphasized that certain social supports can protect against depression just as certain social stresses can cause it. Clinical experience with women who have lasting depression after childbirth suggests that this is a question which merits further investigation.

The clinical picture of these depressions of moderate severity takes the form of a neurotic or asthenic depressive syndrome. Tiredness, anxiety, and irritability are often more prominent than depressive mood change. The clinical picture is not obviously different between those of early onset (in which a relation to changes in female hormones is most plausible) and those which begin late. Prolonged thyroid disorder has been suggested as a cause of these asthenic depressive states, but without any satisfactory evidence. Nor is there evidence that thyroid hormones or any other hormonal treatment is effective.

The balance of evidence points to social and psychological causes for these states. However the most important requirement at present is for better clinical description and for efforts to examine the role of measured 'life events' in the origin and course of these disorders.

Conclusion. In order to review a complicated subject within a short compass, this chapter has considered hormonal causes as if their action were independent of psychological and social factors. It is known, however, that psychological stimuli affect the neuroendocrine system. It is also known that the effects of drugs which alter behaviour and emotions are modified by the psychological state of the subject and it is likely that the same might be true of hormones as well. In our own research into post-partum depression we tried to hold constant as many as possible of these social and psychological variables while attempting to examine endocrine factors. This strategy is appropriate for the first steps in research concerned with other questions about endocrine factors in post-partum depression, but at a later stage the interrelationships will have to be examined as well. It is, however, clear that we have not yet reached the point when even the first stage of research is likely to yield useful answers. Before we come back to it there is much to be done in adding to knowledge of individual differences in endocrine readjustments after childbirth, and in describing in a reliable way the separate depressive syndromes in pregnancy and the puerperium. Otherwise we shall be guessing as wildly about hormonal causes of post-partum depression as did Prichard's generation about the circulation of the blood.

References

Bower, W. H. and Altschule, M. D. (1956). *New Engl. J. Med.* 254, 157.

Brown, G. W., Harris, T. O., and Peto J. (1973). *Psychol. Med.* 12, 159.

Burke, C. W. and Roulet, F. (1970). *Br. med. J.* i, 657.

Cope, C. L. (1972). *Adrenal steroids and disease* (2nd edn.) Pitman Medical, London.

Davidson, J. R. T. (1972). *Br. J. Psychiat.* 121, 659.

Gyermark, L., Genther, G., and Fleming, N. (1967). *Int. J. Neuropharmac.* 6, 191.

Hamilton, J. A. (1962). *Post-partum psychiatric problems.* Mosby, St. Louis.

Jansson, B. (1964). *Acta. psychiat. Scand.* Suppl. 172.

Lubin, B., Gardener, S. H., and Roth, A. (1975). *Psychosom. Med.* 37, 136.

Hormones and post-partum depression

Malleson, J. (1953). *Lancet* 2, 158.
Meares, R., Grimwade, J., and Wood, C. (1976). *J. psychosom. Res.* 20, 605.
Nott, P. N., Franklin, M., Armitage, C., and Gelder, M. G. (1976). *Br. J. Psychiat.* 128, 379.
Pitt, B. (1968). *Hosp. Med.* 2, 815.
Prichard, J. C. (1835). *A treatise on insanity.* Sherwood, Gilbert, and Piper, London.
Seager, C. P. (1960). *J. ment. Sci.* 106, 214.
Stengel, E., Zeitlyn, B. B., and Rayner, E. H. (1958). *J. ment. Sci.* 104, 389.
Yalom, I. D., Lunde, D. T., Moos, R. H., and Hamburg, D. A. (1968). *Arch. gen. Psychiat.* 18, 16.

9

Some socio-cultural determinants of psychiatric morbidity associated with childbearing

J. L. COX

Although Esquirol in 1838 had reported that a large number of women with puerperal psychiatric illness were cared for at home, the majority of studies since then have described only those women with a major puerperal psychosis who had been admitted to a mental hospital (see Hamilton 1962). However, in the last decade, childbearing women with disabling neurotic disorders have been described who would not necessarily have been treated by a psychiatrist and whose illness may have occurred not only after the delivery but also during the pregnancy itself (Nilsson and Almgren 1970).

The explanation for this partial neglect of psychiatric disorder during pregnancy is not certain but may include such rational research dilemmas as the lack of brief rating scales of mood validated for pregnant women in addition to the more irrational attitude that pregnant women should be protected from research enquiry until delivery has safely occurred. A preoccupation with childbearing, whether it is regarded as a continuous process or as a hurdle to be over-come (Breen 1975), may have given undue emphasis to the event of delivery and its emotional sequelae rather than to the psychiatric symptoms that may precede it.

The rates for psychiatric morbidity in women attending an antenatal clinic will be determined by several socio-cultural factors such as the varying use of the sick role by pregnant women (McKinlay 1972), the development of maternity services by middle class professionals for the use of middle class women (Milio 1975), and a higher threshold for psychiatric referral for pregnant women than that applied to puerperal women. Thus during pregnancy, for example, caregivers when confronted by a disturbed woman may adopt a 'wait and see' attitude, whereas during the puerperium a more active psychiatric management might be undertaken.

The use of psychiatric case registers for identifying puerperal and pregnant women who have contacted psychiatric services, when combined with obstetric data, can overcome some of the limitations of those studies based on hospital in-patient data alone. One of the other advantages of such studies is that psychiatric data can be obtained for women prior to their pregnancy and that such women may be used as their own controls when determining the relationship between pregnancy itself and psychiatric morbidity (Kendall, Wainwright, Hailey, and Shannon 1976).

An opportunity to examine other socio-cultural factors associated with childbearing occurred during the author's two-year appointment to the Department of Psychiatry at Makerere University in Uganda where it was apparent that several of the local attitudes towards childbearing contrasted markedly with those found in contemporary Western societies. Only rarely for example would Ugandan women acknowledge that their pregnancy was either unwanted or unplanned and in a traditional Ugandan society childbearing was described as that which defined a woman's existence (Roscoe 1911). In other African countries a new-born child was necessary to create the parents (Lambo 1972) and in Senegal the essential function of a woman was to produce children although these pregnant women entered a world of uncertainties and fears (Collomb, Guena, and Diop 1972).

The interest aroused by these cultural contrasts provided some of the initial motivation for undertaking an extensive prospective study of psychiatric morbidity among Ugandan childbearing women and this paper will describe some of the results of this study with particular emphasis on psychiatric morbidity during pregnancy. An outline of the research methodology can be given but a more comprehensive description is available elsewhere (Cox 1978a).

During the pilot interviews with childbearing Ugandan women it became apparent that some questions which would have been appropriate for Western women were meaningless for the Ganda women being studied. A detailed enquiry about the relationship between a pregnant woman and her mother for example was not appropriate for a society with an extended family system in which the 'mother' role could be shared with aunts and co-wives. Likewise, enquiry about the desirability or planning of the pregnancy would not have been understood by the majority of the 263 women studied and so was omitted from the interview schedule.

Further difficulties encountered included the correct use of interpreters, cultural variants of the sick role, and the reliability of translation. Such difficulties however may occur in *any* study in which the researcher comes from a different ethnic background to the subjects being studied or in which the sample women are ethnically heterogeneous.

In Uganda much of this vital preliminary work had already been carried out by Orley (1973) who had made a detailed study of neurotic symptoms among the Ganda tribe and had translated the Present State Examination (Wing, Cooper, and Sartorius 1974) into the vernacular. However in this study a shorter questionnaire was required which would permit the identification, with an interpreter, of neurotic symptoms. The Standardised Interview Schedule (S.I.S.) (Goldberg, Cooper, Eastwood, Kedward, and Shepherd 1970) was therefore more suitable for this study since both compulsory and probing questions were asked in order to establish the presence or absence of ten defined psychiatric symptoms. This standardized clinical interview allowed flexibility of interview style without reducing reliability. In addition twelve manifest abnormalities of the mental state were rated according to their severity, as described in the interview manual.

The study thus consisted of a psychiatric evaluation of 263 pregnant Ugandan women, who had attended an antenatal clinic at a semi-rural health centre for the first time in their present pregnancy. When possible, such women were followed through to the puerperium for a second interview by the author who again used the S.I.S. In addition 89 non-pregnant and non-puerperal women were interviewed and matched for age, parity, domicile, and marital status with women from the pregnant sample.

The selection of a suitable control group of non-child-bearing women in any culture is a complicated task and among the Ganda this task was made particularly difficult because of the stigma associated with women who were either single or infertile (Bennett 1965). It was decided therefore to select the control group of non-pregnant, non-puerperal women from among those women who attended the general morbidity clinic at the same health centre because of a sick child. It was judged that any bias due to excessive worries among such women would be against the hypothesis that pregnant women had more psychiatric morbidity than non-pregnant, non-puerperal women. The pregnant women were generally representative of Ganda women although their access to the superior medical facilities of the health centre reduced the frequency of complications due to physical illness or obstetric factors.

The psychiatric morbidity of pregnant and control women was evaluated by an analysis of the mean individual scores for the defined psychiatric symptoms, the mean overall severity score, and the clinical evaluation of psychiatric morbidity. The criteria used for the clinical evaluation were as follows:

Certain psychiatric morbidity was said to be present when, in the previous seven days, many psychiatric symptoms were reported which were both socially disabling and also associated with manifest abnormalities of the mental state.

A rating of *uncertain* psychiatric morbidity was made in women whose apparent psychogenic symptoms *could* be explained by a co-existing physical illness, women advanced in pregnancy whose symptoms could not be stated confidently as being in excess of the normal expected for that stage of pregnancy, and women with definite psychiatric symptoms but no evidence of any manifest abnormality of the mental state.

When very few or no symptoms were reported and there

was no abnormality of the mental state, no psychiatric morbidity was recorded.

Certain psychiatric morbidity was found to be present in 16·9 per cent of the pregnant women and in 7·9 per cent of the control sample (Table 9.1). This difference indicated a

Table 9.1. *Comparison of psychiatric morbidity in pregnant and control women* (N = 89 *in each group*)

Psychiatric morbidity	Pregnant sample		Control sample	
	N	per cent	N	per cent
Certain	15	16·9	7	7·9
Uncertain	8	9·0	4	4·5
No morbidity	66	74·2	78	87·6

trend towards increased psychiatric morbidity in pregnant women but did not reach statistical significance unless the certain and uncertain categories of psychiatric morbidity were combined. However a comparison of the mean overall severity scores for the control and pregnant samples did show a highly significant difference ($p < 0.01$, Mann–Whitney U Test).

Comparison of the mean scores for individual symptoms in the pregnant and control samples also showed a significant difference for anxiety but not for depression (Fig. 8). A diagnosis of depression was made in 11·7 per cent of pregnant women and in 6·5 per cent of the non-pregnant, non-puerperal women, whilst an anxiety neurosis was found in 6·5 per cent of the pregnant women but only in 2·6 per cent of the controls.

These findings thus show that pregnant women at their first antenatal attendance experienced more psychiatric symptoms in the preceding week than non-childbearing women and that this difference remained when marital status, parity, age, and domicile were controlled for.

The finding of 16·9 per cent of pregnant women having certain psychiatric morbidity is similar to that of Assael,

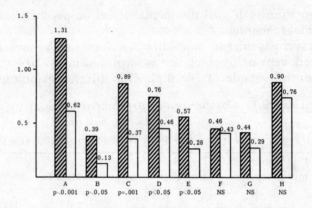

FIG. 8. Comparison of mean ratings of individual symptoms for pregnant (▨) and control (▢) samples. Key to symptoms: (A) subjective evaluation of health; (B) excessive concern with bodily functions; (C) fatigue; (D) anxiety symptom; (E) anxiety observed; (F) depression symptom; (G) depression observed; (H) psychogenic somatic symptoms.

Namboze, German, and Bennett (1972) who found that 24 per cent of pregnant women at Kasangati Health Centre had conspicuous psychiatric morbidity. However no association was found between antenatal psychiatric morbidity and being a co-wife, although pregnant women who were separated from their husbands *were* more likely than other women to have certain psychiatric morbidity (χ^2 = 6·93, 1 d.f., $p < 0·01$).

No association was found between antenatal psychiatric morbidity and age of the women, gravidity, or the length of stay in the defined research area.

Of the 186 women followed to the puerperium 9·7 per cent had a puerperal depression. Thus one of the main findings of the study is that the 'colonial' hypothesis that childbearing in African women is 'natural' and trouble free has received no support and indeed the frequency of puerperal depression seemed surprisingly comparable with that found in London women (Pitt 1968).

It is apparent that an adequate understanding of these results would necessitate an appreciation of relevant sociocultural factors, since childbearing cannot be isolated from the socio-cultural environment in which it occurs. The reasons for the association found between marital separation and psychiatric morbidity for example would necessitate a detailed appreciation of the status of separated Baganda women and also an understanding of the marriage contract in a polygamous patriarchal society. Likewise the explanation for the finding that higher rates of psychiatric morbidity were found in pregnant women than in the control sample would again suggest the need for further studies of the specific stresses associated with pregnancy.

Traditional medicines were taken by 61 per cent of the antenatal sample. These medicines usually consisted of a sausage-shaped lump of clay which was rubbed on to the abdomen or taken as a drink and which was believed to prevent a variety of illnesses and misfortunes which could occur to the childbearing women including the traditional puerperal illness called 'Amakiro'. It is possible that some of the sample women may have received treatment from traditional healers for this illness which has some similarities to Western puerperal psychoses (Cox 1978b). If this did occur, then this could explain the absence from the study of any women known to have an organic or schizophrenic psychosis.

This study has shown that an understanding of some socio-cultural factors is a *sine qua non* if psychiatric morbidity among childbearing Ugandan women is to be fully understood and it seems likely that this perspective is also of importance when considering those mental illnesses which occur in childbearing European women. Thus when searching for the explanation for the increased rates of psychiatric disturbance associated with childbearing in African and European women a knowledge of local beliefs, the availability of traditional remedies, and the reasons for choosing a healer may need to be considered in addition to biological factors.

References

Assael, M. I., Namboze, J. M., German, G. A., and Bennett, F. J. (1972). *Soc. Sci. Med.* **6**, 387.

Bennett, F. J. (1965), *Fertil. Steril.* 16, 243.

Breen, D. (1975). *The birth of a first child.* Tavistock Publications, London.

Collomb, H., Guena, R., and Diop, B. (1972). *Foreign Psychiat.* 1, 77.

Cox, J. L. (1978a). *Psychiatric morbidity and childbearing; a study of 263 semi-rural Ugandan women.* D.M. Thesis Oxford University.

Cox, J. L. (1978b). *Amakiro: a Ugandan puerperal psychosiss? Soc. Psychiat.* in press.

Esquirol, J. E. D. (1838). *Des maladies mentales considérées sous les rapports medical, hygiénique, et médico-légal.* Baillière, Paris.

Goldberg, D. P., Cooper, B., Eastwood, M. R., Kedward, H. B., and Shepherd, M. (1970). *Br. J. prev. soc. Med.* 24, 18.

Hamilton, J. A. (1962). *Post-partum psychiatric disorders.* Mosby, St. Louis.

Kendell, R. E., Wainwright, S., Hailey, A., and Shannon, B. (1976). *Psychol. Med.* 6, 297.

Lambo, T. A. (1972). *Totus Homo* 4, 8.

McKinlay, J. B. (1972). *Soc. Sci. Med.* 6, 561.

Milio, N. (1975). In *A sociology of medical sciences* (ed. C. Cox and A. Mead), pp. 368–88. Collier–Macmillan, London.

Nilsson, A. and Almgren, P. E. (1970). *Acta psychiat. Scand. Suppl.* 220.

Orley, J. H. (1973). *Culture and mental illness in Africa.* D.M. Thesis, Oxford University.

Pitt, B. (1968). *Br. J. Psychiat.* 114, 1325.

Roscoe, J. (1911). *The Baganda—an account of their native customs and beliefs.* Macmillan and Co., London.

Wing, J. K., Cooper, J. E., and Sartorius, N. (1974). *Measurement and classification of psychiatric symptoms.* Cambridge University Press.

10

The effect of psychotropic
drugs on the foetus

P. J. LEWIS

In an ideal world no patient would be exposed to any drug
without the prescriber making careful calculation of the
likely risks and benefits of such an exposure, the calculation
being based on a precise diagnosis and a knowledge of the
drug's efficacy and therapeutic index in that context. Practising physicians will know how far short of this ideal most of
today's clinical practice falls; drugs are easy to prescribe and
both the clinician and the patient are easily attracted by the
idea that some positive action is being taken. Spurious
reasons for drug prescription often outweigh legitimate considerations of the medical and pharmacological factors involved. One consequence of our casual attitude to potent
drugs is the prevalence of iatrogenic complications. No-one
could deny that some adverse reactions to drugs are inevit-
able; they are the price we have to pay for having active
treatments. Nevertheless many adverse reactions arise during
drug exposures which are unnecessary and thus stem from
failure on the part of the clinician to think carefully about
the likely risks and benefits of his actions.

The exposure of pregnant women to psychotropic drugs
presents a particularly delicate dilemma of benefits and
risks (Mirkin 1976a). Other authors in this volume have
described various psychiatric problems which are associated
with pregnancy; they may have argued a case for the potential benefits of treating these complications with psychotropic drugs. In this review I intend to discuss the risks which
the drug-exposed foetus has to take on behalf of its mother.
I shall first review the magnitude of this problem, the extent
to which the human foetus is exposed to psychotropic drugs,

and how these drugs gain access to the foetus. I shall then discuss some possible consequences of such exposure.

Exposure of pregnant women to psychotropic drugs. We live in a highly medicine-ridden society which has a ready acceptance of prescribed drugs, non-prescription drugs, and even illegal drugs. Several surveys have shown that pregnant women are commonly exposed to drugs. Nelson and Forfar (1971) studied drug exposure during pregnancy, but excluding labour, in 1369 women in Scotland. Ninety-seven per cent of these women took prescribed drugs and 65 per cent took over-the-counter drugs. The average number of products taken was two during the first trimester and three and a half during the whole pregnancy. A study of prescriptions given to 457 pregnant Swedish women (Boethius 1977) showed that pregnant women consumed more drugs while they were pregnant than did matched non-pregnant controls. The average number of prescription drugs taken during pregnancy was 3·1.

Figures from the Collaborative Perinatal Project (Heinonen, Slone, and Shapiro 1977) documented drug exposure in 51 282 pregnancies in the U.S.A. between 1959 and 1965. Only 5·8 per cent of these pregnant women had no exposure to drugs during pregnancy. The mean exposure was 3·8 pharmaceutical products per pregnancy. Prescription drugs outnumber non-prescription drugs in most surveys. Pregnant women are aware of the dangers of drugs taken during pregnancy (Baric and MacArthur 1977) and these exposure rates are mainly dependent on physicians' practice and not on the patient.

Psychotropic drugs, by which I shall mean sedatives, tranquillizers, antidepressants, and antipsychotics, form the fourth largest group of drugs taken by women in pregnancy. In the American study just referred to, 35·7 per cent of women took them at some stage of pregnancy. The figures for the critical first trimester were as follows: phenothiazines 2·6 per cent, barbiturates 4·8 per cent, tranquillizers and non-barbiturate sedatives 1·9 per cent, antidepressants 0·1 per cent. Similar exposure rates for psychotropics were reported in the Scottish study. In the Swedish study, psychotropics were taken by 10 per cent of women during pregnancy. These high exposure rates, especially in the first trimester, are somewhat disquieting. It is of particular interest that most of these drugs are not prescribed for the treatment of affective or psychotic disorders. Phenothiazines are employed mainly to treat nausea in early pregnancy; barbiturates are used by obstetricians as a treatment for raised blood pressure in pregnancy. Tricylic antidepressants are perhaps a better index of specific psychoactive therapy and total pregnancy exposure in the American study was only 0·3 per cent of the sample.

The placenta and accessibility of the foetus to drugs. Prior to the thalidomide tragedy in 1959–61, it was widely assumed that the placenta constitutes a selective barrier protecting the foetus from exposure to drugs taken by the mother. Some vestiges of this idea remain with us. Clinicians very commonly ask whether a particular drug 'crosses the placental barrier'. A concise answer to this question is that all drugs penetrate the placenta but their rate of penetration varies very widely (Mirkin 1976b). Some drugs which are very highly ionized, such as heparin or the skeletal muscle relaxants, penetrate the placenta extremely slowly. However, the majority of drugs rapidly equilibrate wih foetal tissues. Lipophilicity determines the speed of placental transfer and since all psychotropic drugs are lipophilic, or they would not penetrate the central nervous system, psychotropic drugs all gain access to the foetus.

The distribution of drug within the foetus may differ from that in the adult for a variety of reasons. Foetal plasma protein binds drugs less strongly than does adult plasma protein and hence tissue to blood ratios in the foetus may be higher than in the adult. Since a greater proportion of foetal cardiac output is directed towards the brain than in the adult, the foetal brain is more rapidly exposed to any drug diffusing across the placenta.

101

The effect of psychotropic drugs on the foetus

Acute pharmacological effects on the foetus. The majority of psychotropic drugs are depressants of the central nervous system. This is particularly evident when they are given in large doses to immature individuals. Depression of the central nervous system in the neonate, as evidenced by somnolence, failure to establish spontaneous respiration, poor feeding, and hypothermia, is a common consequence of maternal treatment during delivery with central-acting drugs. In most cases the drugs are analgesics and anaesthetic compounds. But psychotropics such as diazepam or phenothiazines are also used during labour, either as anxiolytics or as anticonvulsants in women with raised arterial pressure. Two main factors tend to exacerbate these central nervous depressant effects of drugs given during labour on the neonate. The first is the pharmacokinetic factor mentioned previously. If the drug is given intravenously to the mother resulting in high peak plasma concentrations, then after a short period of time the foetal blood drug concentration will exceed that of maternal plasma and the foetus will have a persistently high concentration of drug. The second factor is the relatively poor ability of the neonate to eliminate drugs by metabolism (Murdock, Thorgeirsson, Rossiger, and Davies 1975). This leads to persistence of pharmacologically significant levels of drug in the neonate (Cooper, Stephen, and Aggett 1977).

Studies with the benzodiazepine, diazepam, illustrate these considerations. The cord blood concentration of diazepam is generally higher than that in maternal blood (Scher, Hailey, and Beard 1972). Central nervous system depression in neonates exposed to diazepam during labour is very common, especially when large doses have been used, as is usual for the treatment of pre-eclampsia. Diazepam impairs temperature regulation in the neonate (Owen, Irani, and Blair 1972) and after large doses of the drug, diazepam can be detected in the neonatal serum until the seventh day of life (McCarthy, O'Connell, and Robinson 1973). It has been recommended that mothers in labour should not be given more than 20 mg diazepam because of its depressant effect on the foetus (Kanto, Erkkola, and Sellman 1974).

Prolonged depression of the neonates of women on

102

chronic treatment with chlorpromazine has been reported and an extrapyramidal syndrome has been reported in an infant born to a mother treated with this drug (Hill, Desmond, and Kay 1966). Irritability and depression in the neonate have been reported after delivery in women who have taken imipramine throughout pregnancy (Eggermont, Raveschot, Deneve, and Casteels-Van Deele 1972).

These central effects of psychotropic drugs on the foetus are obviously of most practical importance in the perinatal period. However, it is now possible to document similar depressive effects of psychotropic drugs during pregnancy using ultrasound. Large doses of pethidine and diazepam have been reported to inhibit foetal breathing *in utero* (Boddy 1977). Foetal breathing is thought to be a subtle indicator of central nervous system arousal in the foetus and in animal experiments it can be depressed with psychotropic drugs (Piercy, Day, Neims, and Williams 1977). However, the human foetus does not seem to be particularly sensitive to these drugs and small doses of pethidine and diazepam do not have a measurable effect on the frequency of intra-uterine breathing movements (unpublished observations).

Teratogenicity. There is no compelling evidence that psychotropic drugs exert teratogenic effects in man. However, the methods available to assign different drugs to various risk categories for human teratogenicity are acknowledged to be very unsatisfactory, relying as they do on epidemiological studies of great administrative complexity which are subject to biased reporting on the part of mothers with congenitally abnormal children. Nevertheless a consensus has arisen which categorizes different drugs in order of teratogenic suspicion (Wilson 1973). Currently accepted as probably teratogenic in man are oestrogens, tetracycline, phenytoin (and probably other anticonvulsants), and folic acid antagonists.

Animal experiments are of limited value in predicting teratogenic potential in man and are mainly carried out in order to satisfy drug regulatory authorities (Robson 1970). However, for what it is worth, psychotropic agents show low teratogenic potency in animals. No antidepressant drugs are teratogenic in mice; some are teratogenic in rats and rabbits. Only one monoamine oxidase inhibitor, phenelzine, is teratogenic in the rat. Phenothiazine and butyrophenone antipsychotic agents are more teratogenic but of these only trifluoperazine is active in rabbits. Anxiolytics have low teratogenicity scores but diazepam produces similar lesions in rats to those produced by the known human teratogen, phenytoin (Miller and Becker 1975). However, the doses required are larger.

So far as human pregnancy is concerned almost all psychoactive drugs have been associated in isolated case reports with the production of abnormalities but there are few epidemiological series to confirm these associations (Schardein 1976). A recent prospective study by the French National Institute of Health and Medical Research included 12 764 women. Amongst the 189 who gave birth to babies with non-chromosomal-based malformations, there was a significant excess of women who had taken phenothiazines during the first three months of pregnancy (Rumeau-Roquette, Goujard, and Huel 1977). The phenothiazine-associated abnormalities were very varied, ranging from multiple skeletal malformations through to cleft lip and palate. It is of interest that of these 11 women prescribed phenothiazines in early pregnancy, none was thought to be psychotic; the indications for prescription included insomnia, vomiting, depression, and allergy.

Saxen (1975) investigated the foetal history of 599 children with oral clefts using the Finnish register of congenital malformations. During the first trimester of these affected pregnancies, the consumption of antineurotic drugs, mainly diazepam, was twice that in matched control pregnancies, 6·2 versus 2·99 per cent. A similar association of diazepam with cleft palate has been reported from Norway (Aarskog 1975). Data from the U.S. Collaborative Perinatal Project correlating drug consumption in 50 282 pregnancies to congenital abnormality show a slight excess of abnormal children born to these women exposed to sedatives, tranquillizers, or antidepressants during the first trimester of pregnancy. This excess was very small and only just achieved statistical significance for the group as a whole. there was no excess risk found for women exposed to phenothiazines in the first trimester of pregnancy.

Enzyme induction. Many different chemical substances, when administered to animals, induce the synthesis of microsomal enzymes that metabolize drugs, carcinogens, and endogenous substances such as steroid hormones and bilirubin. Inducing agents include such food substances as the xanthines and flavones, food additives, insecticides, and many drugs (Conney, Welch, Kuntzman, Chang, Jacobsen, Munro-Faure, Peck, Bye, Poland, Poppers, Finster, and Wolff 1971). Thus, apart from their immediate pharmacological effect, psychotropics may also exert long-term effects by influencing the activity of enzyme systems within the body. Such an effect may also be exerted on enzyme systems developing within the foetus (Sereni, Mandelli, Princip, Tognoni, Pardi, and Morselli 1973).

It is established that hepatic microsomal drug-metabolizing enzymes are poorly developed in foetal and new-born laboratory animals. The development of drug-metabolizing capacity in the human foetus is also though to be slow and the human neonate metabolizes drug substances at one-half to one-quarter of the adult rate. There is controversy as to whether hepatic microsomal enzyme systems in foetal liver can be induced (i.e. have their activity increased) by exposure to drugs. Animal studies suggest that this can occur (Darby 1971) but there is little information concerning the possibility in the human foetus. Most work has been done on the effect of barbiturates given in late pregnancy on neonatal jaundice. Bilirubin is metabolized in the neonate by conjugation in the liver with glucuronic acid. In neonates treated prenatally with barbiturates, glucuronidation is accelerated and this effect is the basis for their use in the prophylactic treatment of neonatal jaundice (Trolle 1968). However, it is not clear whether this is a true enzyme induction or an effect on bilirubin uptake into the neonatal liver. Sereni *et al.* (1973) demonstrated that in new-borns exposed to phenobarbitone during foetal life, diazepam is more rapidly

105

metabolized than in neonates not so exposed. However, in other studies, neonatal metabolism of amylobarbitone was uninfluenced by prenatal exposure of the foetus to barbiturates (Draffan, Dollery, Davies, Krauer, Williams, Clare, Trudinger, Darling, Sentel, and Hawkins 1976) and neonatal metabolism of cortisol was unaffected by anticonvulsant medication (Reynolds and Mirkin 1973).

Since many psychoactive drugs, including barbiturates and phenothiazines but not benzodiazepines, have activity as inducing agents it is an open possibility that chronic treatment of mothers during pregnancy with these drugs might induce enzyme activity within the foetus.

The consequences of enzyme induction within the foetus are not known (Wilson 1971). However, it has been suggested that the foetus is protected from lipid-soluble substrates *in utero* by its lack of capacity to metabolize them to more polar substances which would be retained longer within the foetus. Furthermore, alteration of foetal microsomal activity might alter the toxicity of other substances to which the foetus is exposed since metabolites of these substances may be more reactive than their parent species. We know of co-carcinogens; may there not be co-teratogens?

Behavioural teratogenicity. Changes in central nervous activity in the foetus and in the neonate exposed to psychotropic drugs *in utero* have already been discussed. These effects on behaviour are immediate and are due to the direct action of the drug on the foetus. However, animal experiments over the last fifteen years have made it increasingly likely that a prenatally administered drug can influence behaviour in the offspring long after the drug itself has been eliminated. This delayed effect of prenatal drug exposure has been termed behavioural teratogenesis (Coyle, Wayner, and Singer 1976).

The phenothiazine, chlorpromazine, has been one of the drugs most investigated in this regard. Ordy, Samorajski, Collins, and Rolsten (1966) administered chlorpromazine and placebo treatments throughout pregnancy to two groups of mice. At birth the litters were exchanged between treated and non-treated mothers. When tested at 20 and 60 days of age those mice which had received prenatal chlorpromazine performed less well in avoidance tests and explored a smaller area when exposed to an open field situation. Those mice exposed to higher levels of chlorpromazine prenatally were more retarded than those exposed to smaller doses. A similar retardation of behaviour in rats exposed prenatally to chlorpromazine was noted by Clark *et al.* (1970). Similar experiments with amphetamine also produced behavioural retardation in prenatally exposed rats. However, it must be admitted that some authors have failed to find any difference in the behaviour of rats exposed to chlorpromazine or placebo prenatally (Werboff and Havlena 1962). Indeed Golub and Kornetsky (1974) reported that rats treated prenatally with chlorpromazine were in general more active than those not treated and made a more rapid adaptation to avoidance techniques. Some of these discrepancies may be methodological as behavioural teratogenicity is a difficult subject to investigate. Variations in the time of exposure during pregnancy, in the dose of drugs used, in the application of cross-fostering, and in the type of tests of behaviour used all make these investigations difficult to reproduce.

The elegant experiments of Coyle and Singer (1975a) are of particular interest because they illustrate some of the complexities of this work. Rats treated prenatally with the tricyclic antidepressant, imipramine, could not be shown to differ in their behaviour from those treated with placebo provided both groups of rats were housed in a 'deprived' environment. The 'deprived' rats were housed in small boxes lacking any internal features. However, if the experiment was repeated while the rats were housed in large, light boxes in which interesting objects were scattered, such as exercise wheels and so on, then a difference could be shown between those rats treated prenatally with imipramine and those treated with placebo. The imipramine-treated rats performed significantly less well in behavioural tests.

In a further experiment, Coyle and Singer (1975b) demonstrated that placebo-treated rats housed in a 'stimulating' environment developed an optical cerebral cortex which was some 10 per cent thicker than that of similar rats raised in a 'deprived' environment. However, if the rats had been treated prenatally with imipramine, then they showed no difference in cerebral cortex thickness despite being raised in 'stimulating' conditions. This is a most interesting finding; it obviously suggests that rats exposed prenatally to imipramine are unable to react to a stimulating environment and take advantage of the educational opportunities offered them. The experiments also illustrate the subtleties of animal behaviour and the various factors which must be taken into account when designing these complicated experiments.

Other drugs which have been shown to exert behavioural teratogenic effects include meprobamate, reserpine, barbiturates, amphetamine, cannabis, and methyl mercury. The biochemical basis for behavioural teratogenesis is fairly straightforward; interference with neurotransmitter synthesis, release, or function may interfere with the physical development of interneuronal connections within the CNS. Such effects have been demonstrated in the autonomic nervous system (Bartholomé and Slotkin 1976).

What implications do these experiments have for human children exposed *in utero* to centrally acting drugs? So far as I am aware there are only two instances of behavioural teratogenicity in man. The first is a very gross case, Minimata disease, or methyl mercury poisoning. Japanese children exposed to this pollutant *in utero* as a result of their mothers eating fish contaminated with methyl mercury show no overt morphological abnormality but they have a variety of neurological disorders and most are mentally retarded. This may be regarded as a gross form of behavioural teratogenicity.

The other example in man is that of smoking. The follow-up study of Butler and Goldstein (1973) on the offspring of women who smoked during the latter five months of pregnancy included educational tests on children at the age of 11. There was a significant retardation in reading age in the children whose mothers had smoked during their pregnancy compared with the children of mothers who did not smoke, even when the results were corrected for social class. This is a more subtle form of behavioural teratogenicity and is of the type we might anticipate as being caused by psychotropic drug exposure *in utero.*

If behavioural changes are induced in children exposed to psychotropic drugs prenatally, this will be very difficult to detect. Human behaviour is extremely plastic; postnatal social and parental influences are so dominant that it would seem extremely unlikely that any subtle form of behaviour change could be detected without a very considerable research effort, testing many exposed children and a comparable control group. The confounding influences of education, opportunity, and social class are obvious pitfalls. The possibility of behavioural teratogenicity in human beings caused by psychotropic drugs will probably remain unproven, but animal studies do suggest that the developing central nervous system is susceptible to these drug effects. In human beings, brain development extends over the whole of pregnancy and into early neonatal life and hence vulnerability to such effects must be extended similarly.

This is a brief general review of four potential risks to the foetus when exposed *in utero* to psychotropic drugs. It is only fair to point out that, in discussing each of these four adverse consequences of exposure, little hard data can be brought forward to convince sceptics that these effects are produced in practice when the woman takes a course of, for example, diazepam. These are theoretical risks but I do suggest that their likelihood must be weighed against the possible benefits of treatment. As rational prescribers, we can accept big risks if drugs are very important. We do this in pregnancy with the very much more sinister hydantoin anticonvulsants. I would suggest, however, that for the treatment of neurotic conditions which resolved spontaneously, we cannot accept anything but trivial risk.

References

Aarskog, D. (1975). *Lancet* ii, 921.
Baric, L. and MacArthur, C. (1977). *Br. J. prev. soc. Med.* 31, 30.
Bartholomé, J. and Slotkin, T. A. (1976). *Biochem. Pharmac.* 25, 1513

The effect of psychotropic drugs on the foetus

Boethius, G. (1977). *Eur. J. clin. Pharmac.* 72, 37.

Boddy, K. (1977). In *Therapeutic problems in pregnancy* (ed. P. J. Lewis), p. 153. Medical and Technical Press, Lancaster.

Butler, N. R. and Goldstein, H. (1973). *Br. med. J.* ii, 573.

Clark, C. V. H., Gorman, D., and Vernadakis, A. (1970). *Devel. Psychobiol.* 3, 225.

Conney, A. H., Welch, R., Kuntzman, R., Chang, R., Jacobsen, M., Munro-Faure, A. D., Peck, A. W., Bye, A., Poland, A., Poppers, P. J., Finster, M., and Wolff, J. A. (1971). *Ann. N.Y. Acad. Sci.* 179, 155.

Cooper, L. V., Stephen, G. W., and Aggett, P. J. A. (1977). *Arch. Dis. Childh.* 52, 638.

Coyle, I. R. and Singer, G. (1975a). *Psychopharmacologia* 41, 237.

—— — (1975b). *Psychopharmacologia* 44, 253.

—— Wayner, M. J., and Singer, G. (1976). *Pharmac. Biochem. Behav.* 4, 191.

Darby, F. J. (1971). *Biochem. J.* 122, 41.

Draffan, G. H., Dollery, C. T., Davies, D. S., Krauer, B., Williams, F. M., Clare, R. A., Trudinger, B. J., Darling, M., Sertel, M., and Hawkins, D. F. (1976). *Clin. Pharmac. Ther.* 19, 271.

Eggermont, E., Raveschot, J., Deneve, V., and Casteels-Van Deele, M. (1972). *Acta Pediat. Belg.* 26, 197.

Golub, M. and Kornetsky, C. (1974). *Devel. Psychobiol.* 7, 79.

Heinonen, O. P., Slone, D., and Shapiro, S. (1977). In *Birth defects and drugs in pregnancy.* Publishing Sciences Group, Boston, Massachusetts.

Hill, R. M., Desmond, M. M., and Kay, J. L. (1966). *J. Pediat.* 69, 589.

Kanto, J., Erkkola, R., and Sellman, R. (1974). *Br. med. J.* i, 641.

McCarthy, G. T., O'Connell, B., and Robinson, A. E. (1973). *J. Obstet. Gynaec. Brit. Comm.* 80, 349.

Miller, R. P. and Becker, B. A. (1975). *Toxicol. Appl. Pharmac.* 32, 53.

Mirkin, B. L. (1976a). *Clin. Toxicol.* 9, 93.

— (1976b). *Pediat. Ann.* 5, 542.

Murdock, A. I., Thorgeirsson, S. S., Rossiger, H., and Davies, D. S. (1975). *Biol. Neonate* 27, 289.

Nelson, M. M. and Forfar, J. O. (1971). *Br. med. J.* i, 523.

Ordy, J. M., Samorajski, T., Collins, R. L., and Rolsten, C. (1966). *J. Pharmac. exp. Ther.* 151, 110.

Owen, J. R., Irani, S. F., and Blair, A. W. (1972). *Arch. Dis. Childh.* 47, 107.

Piercy, W. N., Day, M. A., Neims, A. H., and Williams, R. L. (1977). *Am. J. Obstet. Gynec.* 127, 43.

Reynolds, J. W. and Mirkin, B. L. (1973). *Clin. Pharmac. Ther.* 14, 891.

Robson, J. M. (1970). *Br. med. Bull.* 26, 212.

Rumeau-Rouquette, C., Goujard, J., and Huel, G. (1977). *Teratology* 15, 57.

The effect of psychotropic drugs on the foetus

Saxen, I. (1975). *Int. J. Epidemiol.* 4, 37.

Schardein, J. L. (1976). *Drugs as teratogens.* CRC Press, Cleveland, Ohio.

Scher, J., Hailey, D.M., and Beard, R. W. (1972). *J. Obstet. Gynaec. Brit. Comm.* 79, 635.

Sereni, F., Mandelli, M., Princip, N., Tognoni, G., Pardi, G., and Morselli, P. L. (1973). *Enzyme* 15, 318.

Trolle, D. (1968). *Lancet* ii, 705.

Werboff, J. and Havlena, J. (1962). *Exp. Neurol.* 6, 263.

Wilson, J. T. (1971). *Clin. Pediat.* 10, 684.

Wilson, J. G. (1973). *Teratology* 7, 3.

11

Maternal mental illness – the effect on the baby

DAVID HARVEY

Mothers with mental illness, particularly neurotic disorders, cause a lot of concern to paediatricians because they often bring their babies to clinics with feeding or sleeping problems. A number of studies have shown that children who attend child guidance clinics are more likely to have parents with psychiatric disorders than other children (Rutter 1966). Clearly, there seems to be a relationship between emotional problems in the child and mental illness in the mother. Here we are concerned with the young baby. Many of them do not seem to suffer long-term consequences even when the mother has a severe psychosis, but there does appear to be a greater chance of injury and death. Paediatricians are familiar with the many babies brought to out-patient departments or child health centres where the baby's problem seems closely related to neurotic disorders in the mother. It is common to be presented with a baby who cries incessantly, vomits often, refuses feeds, or does not sleep. Very often the mother seems to be the one who is unwell. She seems pathologically depressed or anxious.

Puerperal psychosis. Some studies have suggested that there is a relationship between puerperal psychosis and abnormalities in the baby at the time of birth. Paffenbarger's (1964) work has been mentioned more than once in this context. Women with pre-partum or post-partum mental illness were compared with a control group of women. There was evidence that the duration of gestation is shorter in women with post-partum mental illness: the mean gestational age in 68 babies of mothers with pre-partum mental illness was

39·5 weeks, compared with 39·1 weeks in 232 babies of women with post-partum mental illness and 39·6 weeks in 616 babies of control women. The mean gestational age was significantly lower in the post-partum mental illness group ($p < 0.05$). The shortened period of gestation was reflected in the mean birth weight of the babies. That of the babies of women mentally ill after delivery was 150 g lower than the control group or 175 g lower after allowing for maternal age and parity. The mean birth weight was 3320 g in the control group and 3154 g in the post-partum group.

The same study suggested that there was also an increased incidence of abnormalities in labour and a greater risk of peri-natal mortality. There was a history of maternal dystocia in 26 out of 242 infants in the post-partum group (11 per cent), but in only 35 out of 628 infants in the control group (6 per cent). The perinatal mortality was higher in the post-partum group at six per thousand, compared with three per thousand in the control group. The figures for dystocia and perinatal mortality are significantly less in the post-partum group than in the control group ($p < 0.05$).

It is difficult to be certain whether these differences are cause or effect. It is quite conceivable that mental illness appeared more frequently in women who had a difficult labour or who had lost their babies.

Pregnancy in patients with neuroses. There is also evidence that disorders of pregnancy and death of the baby at birth are commoner in patients with neurotic illness. Bahna and Bjerkedal (1974) studied 388 pregnancies in women with neuroses and compared them with a control group of 112 532 pregnancies in other women. Some results of their study are shown in Table 12.1.

The difference in the incidence of low birth weight babies between the two groups was significant ($p < 0.001$). It can be seen that, in all the items mentioned, the neurotic group were worse. They had shorter gestation, more small babies, the babies were more likely to be ill or to die, and interven-tion was needed in labour more often. These factors are often used as indices of health in pregnancy. Therefore, it seems

Table 12.1. *Problems of pregnancies in patients with neurosis (taken from Bahna and Bjerkedal 1974)*

	Neurosis group $n = 388$	Control group $n = 112\ 532$	
Mean gestation	39·2 weeks	39·9 weeks	
Percentage of low-birth weight babies	8·5	3·7	$p < 0·001$
Babies with malformation, disease, or birth injury (per cent)	10·9	3·9	
Perinatal mortality rate (per 1000)	35·7	14·6	
Intervention needed (per cent)	18	7·7	

that these women are at high risk and need careful attention during pregnancy and labour for their babies' sakes.

Risk of injury or death to the baby after birth. Perhaps the problem that concerns us most is infanticide; we are also worried by a disordered relationship between a mother and her child, which could easily lead to injury. Seager (1960) reported one case of infanticide in 42 patients with post-partum mental illness. It was interesting that the author reported that six patients at follow-up still blamed the child for the mental illness; two of them wished to harm the baby. One mother had the interesting symptom that she had lost her love for the baby, but the love later returned. Ryle (1961) also reported patients who had lost their love for their babies.

There has been a lot of interest recently in the battered baby syndrome, which is also called non-accidental injury. It seems that some parents who injure their children are mentally ill and others have been disturbed by events around the time of childbirth. Smith (1975) studied the parents of 125 children with the battered child syndrome and compared them with the parents of a control group of children who had entered hospital for other illnesses. He observed psychotic reactions in four mothers (3·2 per cent of the mothers) and one father. Two of the mothers were paranoid schizophrenics and one had killed her two children. Two other mothers were psychotically depressed. One very interesting finding, which may be helpful in clinical practice, is that the injuries inflicted by psychotic parents were extremely bizarre. Very unusual injuries should therefore immediately indicate that the parents should be investigated for mental disturbance. Smith also studied the incidence of neurotic disorders in the parents of these children. The results are shown in Table 12.2. It is clear that the index group (mothers of battered children) showed a much higher incidence of neurotic disturbances. Thirty-four of these mothers showed mixed neurotic symptomatology, 21 were depressed, two showed anxiety reactions, and two had hysterical reactions. One patient was agoraphobic and another had anorexia nervosa.

These findings should alert us when we see pregnant women with neurotic disorders. They will probably need a lot of support in caring for their children. It is important not to do anything in the hospital which might increase the risk of non-accidental injury. Recently, it has become clear that one of the worst things we can do is admit a baby to the special care unit and separate him from his mother. There are of course many good reasons why babies should be admitted to the special care unit, for instance if they are very small or need special nursing. Unfortunately, large babies in recent years have been observed in the special care unit after a difficult delivery; this unnecessary time of separation has now been stopped in most units. Lynch and Roberts (1977) looked at 50 babies with non-accidental injuries and compared them with 50 controls. In the non-accidental-injury group 21 (42 per cent) had been admitted to a special care unit compared with 5 (10 per cent) in the control group. This interesting observation was confirmed by studying other non-accidental-injury patients with their siblings. Enquiries

Table 12.2. *Neurotic features in parents of children with the battered child syndrome (taken from Smith 1975)*

	Non-neurotic		Neurotic	
	Number	Per cent	Number	Per cent
Mothers of children with battered-child syndrome	65	52	60	48
Mothers of control children	40	90	5	10

were made about 25 children with non-accidental injury; of these, 10 (40 per cent) had been separated from their mothers in the new-born period and 9 (36 per cent) had some other separation early in life. The history in 35 siblings was quite different; none of them had been injured by their parents. Only two out of 35 (6 per cent) had had neonatal separation and two (6 per cent) had some other separation.

We have learnt recently that closeness of contact between the mother and baby in the first day or two after delivery has long-lasting results (Klaus and Kennell 1976). For instance, different behaviour in the mother and baby has been observed throughout the first two years when there has been a time of skin-to-skin contact in the new-born period between a naked baby and his mother. The mother appears later to be more loving towards her baby and he responds more to her. These studies have important lessons for those of us who work in maternity hospitals.

Depression in young mothers. Not only does separation in early life lead to a greater risk of being injured by one's parents, but the child when he or she becomes a parent seems to have a higher incidence of depression and of difficulties in rearing young children. It would be extremely useful if we could tell before delivery which women were more likely to present in baby clinics with baby problems. The work of Frommer and O'Shea (1973a) has given us a clue to the antenatal identification of these women. The authors gave a questionnaire to married British primigravidae to find out if any of them had been separated from either or both their parents before the age of 11 years or if either of the parents had died before the woman reached that age. The mother was interviewed antenatally and when the baby was 2–3 months, 6–7 months, 9–10 months, and about 13 months old. There were 40 women in the separated group and they were compared with 30 women who did not report separation. There did not appear to be many differences during pregnancy apart from the incidence of major depression. Ten women in each group (25 per cent of the separated group and 33 per cent of the non-separated group) showed anxiety about the pregnancy and minor depression was present in 16 (40 per cent) of the separated women and 15 (50 per cent) of the non-separated women. The major difference was that twice as many women who had been separated from parents before the age of 11 had major depression (8, or 20 per cent, of the separated group compared with 3, or 10 per cent, of the non-separated group).

In the follow-up of these children, it became clear that depression was much commoner during the first year after birth in the women in the separated group. At the fourth postnatal visit when the child was about 13 months of age, 29 of the separated women reported depression or appeared depressed to the observer—this is 64 per cent of the whole group. Depression was only present in 15 (34 per cent) of the non-separated group and the result is significantly different ($p < 0.05$).

This frightening result is very important to those working with mothers and young children. What is interesting to a paediatrician is that the babies were more likely to have feeding or sleeping problems. For instance, the total number of feeding problems in the first year in the separated group was 19 minor problems (41 per cent) and 8 major problems (17 per cent). This can be compared with 8 minor problems (18 per cent) and 2 major problems (5 per cent) in the non-separated group. The difference in the incidence of minor problems is significant ($p < 0.05$). At the second postnatal visit there was a significant difference in the number of major

117

sleeping problems reported in the babies. Nine of the separated women reported that their baby had this problem (20 per cent) and only 2 of the other group (4 per cent). Again, this is significant ($p < 0.05$). Of course, one cannot be certain whether there were really more problems in the babies or whether they were being reported more frequently by women who were anxious or depressed about the baby. In a sense this is not of great importance, since the problems appear in child health centres and paediatric out-patients, and the mother's illness must be recognized by the paediatrician. The doctor must not concentrate on the baby, but look on the baby as a member of the family who might have problems.

In another paper on the same group of women, Frommer and O'Shea (1973b) looked at a number of factors in women who were classed as having problems in the first year of their infant's life, compared with those who had no problems. Again a history of separation from parents was much commoner in those women who had problems with their babies and there was also very often a history of serious parental quarrelling or a poor relationship with the father. Not surprisingly they found that present marital problems were also associated with baby problems.

These observations are confirmed by other studies which suggest that loss of a mother before 11 years may dispose a young woman to become depressed (Brown, Bhrolcháin, and Harris 1975). It seems that maternal depression and therefore a difficult period for the baby with feeding and sleeping problems is very common in London. Richman (1976) has shown the high incidence of depression in young women. Two studies have suggested that 26 to 40 per cent of women with young children in two London boroughs were depressed. The problem was commonest in young working class women with children under 6 years of age.

It seems that there are at least four vulnerability factors associated with depression; they may help us to pinpoint those women who will have problems:

Lack of a confiding relationship with husband or boyfriend;

Having 3 or more children under the age of 14 years;
Having lost her own mother before the age of 11 years;
and
Not going out to work.

Probably the last is related to isolation in the home. It does seem also that poor housing and little money may be important in producing depression.

Certainly, these problems seem very common to a paediatrician practising in London. It means that we must work much more closely with child psychiatrists to help families with depression who often appear in our clinics.

References

Bahna, S. L. and Bjerkedal, T. (1974). *Acta Obstet. Gynaec. Scand.* 53, 129.

Brown, G. W., Bhrolcháin, N. M., and Harris, T. (1975). *Sociology* 9, 225.

Frommer, E. A. and O'Shea, T. (1973a). *Br. J. Psychiat.* 123, 149.

—— —— (1973b). *Br. J. Psychiat.* 123, 157.

Klaus, M. H. and Kennell, J. H. (1976). *Maternal–infant bonding.* Mosby, St. Louis.

Lynch, M. and Roberts, J. (1977). In *Child abuse, prediction, prevention, and follow-up* (ed. A. W. Franklin). Churchill-Livingstone, Edinburgh.

Paffenbarger, R. S. (1964). *Br. J. prevent. soc. Med.* 18, 189.

Richman, N. (1976). *J. child Psychol. Psychiat.* 17, 75.

Rutter, M. (1966). *Children of sick parents. An environmental and psychiatric study.* Maudsley Monograph No. 16, Oxford University Press, Oxford.

Ryle, A. (1961). *J. ment. Sci.* 101, 279.

Seager, C. P. (1960). *J. ment. Sci.* 106, 214.

Smith, S. M. (1975). *Battered child syndrome.* Butterworth, London.

Index

Index

Index